Service-Learning in Occupational Therapy Education

Philosophy and Practice

Kathleen Flecky, OTD, OTR/L
Assistant Professor
Department of Occupational Therapy
Core Faculty, Office of Interprofessional Scholarship, Service, and Education
School of Pharmacy and Health Professions
Creighton University

Lynn Gitlow, PhD, OTR/L, ATP
Director and Professor
Department of Occupational Therapy
Husson University

JONES AND BARTLETT PUBLISHERS
Sudbury, Massachusetts
BOSTON   TORONTO   LONDON   SINGAPORE

World Headquarters
Jones and Bartlett
  Publishers
40 Tall Pine Drive
Sudbury, MA 01776
978-443-5000
info@jbpub.com
www.jbpub.com

Jones and Bartlett
  Publishers Canada
6339 Ormindale Way
Mississauga, Ontario L5V 1J2
Canada

Jones and Bartlett
  Publishers International
Barb House, Barb Mews
London W6 7PA
United Kingdom

Jones and Bartlett's books and products are available through most bookstores and online booksellers. To contact Jones and Bartlett Publishers directly, call 800-832-0034, fax 978-443-8000, or visit our website, www.jbpub.com.

Substantial discounts on bulk quantities of Jones and Bartlett's publications are available to corporations, professional associations, and other qualified organizations. For details and specific discount information, contact the special sales department at Jones and Bartlett via the above contact information or send an email to specialsales@jbpub.com.

The authors, editor, and publisher have made every effort to provide accurate information. However, they are not responsible for errors, omissions, or for any outcomes related to the use of the contents of this book and take no responsibility for the use of the products and procedures described. Treatments and side effects described in this book may not be applicable to all people; likewise, some people may require a dose or experience a side effect that is not described herein. Drugs and medical devices are discussed that may have limited availability controlled by the Food and Drug Administration (FDA) for use only in a research study or clinical trial. Research, clinical practice, and government regulations often change the accepted standard in this field. When consideration is being given to use of any drug in the clinical setting, the health care provider or reader is responsible for determining FDA status of the drug, reading the package insert, and reviewing prescribing information for the most up-to-date recommendations on dose, precautions, and contraindications, and determining the appropriate usage for the product. This is especially important in the case of drugs that are new or seldom used.

Production Credits
Publisher: David Cella
Acquisitions Editor: Kristine Jones
Associate Editor: Maro Gartside
Production Director: Amy Rose
Senior Production Editor: Renée Sekerak
Marketing Manager: Grace Richards
Manufacturing and Inventory Control Supervisor:
  Amy Bacus

Cover and Title Page Design: Kate Ternullo
Cover Image: © Jorge Enrique
  Villalobos/ShutterStock, Inc.
Composition: Glyph International
Printing and Binding: Malloy, Incorporated
Cover Printing: Malloy, Incorporated

Library of Congress Cataloging-in-Publication Data
Service-learning in occupational therapy education : philosophy and practice / [edited by] Kathleen Flecky, Lynn Gitlow.
    p. ; cm.
Includes bibliographical references.
ISBN 978-0-7637-5958-2 (alk. paper)
1. Occupational therapy—Study and teaching. 2. Service learning. I. Flecky, Kathleen. II. Gitlow, Lynn.
[DNLM: 1. Occupational Therapy—education. WB 18 S491 2011]
RM735.42.S47 2011
615.8'515—dc22

2009042694

6048

Printed in the United States of America
13 12 11 10 09   10 9 8 7 6 5 4 3 2 1

Contents

**Chapter 3 Who Sits at the Head of the Table?
A Reflection on Community, Student,
and Faculty Partnerships 37**
Beth P. Velde, PhD, OTR/L
Doris T. Davis
Gary R. Grant

**Chapter 4 Cross-Cultural Service-Learning:
An Introduction and Best Practices 59**
Joy D. Doll, OTD, OTR/L

Chapter 10   **Community Engagement: A Process for
Curriculum Integration** **253**
Kimberly Hartmann, PhD, OTR/L, FAOTA

Chapter 11   **Involve Me and I Understand:
Differentiating Service-Learning
and Fieldwork** **275**
Patricia Crist, PhD, OTR, FAOTA

Appendix 11-A Engaged Learning Resources List

Chapter 12 Conclusions and Reflections on Service-Learning in Occupational Therapy Education

Lynn Gitlow, PhD, OTR/L, ATP
Kathleen Flecky, OTD, OTR/L

Preface

"I realized how much occupational therapists can do in the community."
"I feel I know more about what OTs can do rather than just what they do."

These students' reflections on their experiences as part of an occupational therapy service-learning course demonstrate the impact of service-learning on professional formation of students as part of occupational therapy education. *Service-Learning in Occupational Therapy Education: Philosophy and Practice* grew out of our conviction that service-learning can promote the development of core professional formation and skill competencies needed by occupational therapy professionals for occupation-based practice in the twenty-first century (Gitlow & Flecky, 2002).

Since our first joint endeavor in the development of three service-learning courses in 2000, we have been committed to a perspective of professional education as a shared endeavor with community partners to promote students as citizens who move beyond the ability to answer the question: What knowledge and skills do I need to practice occupational therapy in community settings? More importantly, how should I use my knowledge and skills to practice and live in relational communities with others as agents for social change? Our research and writings have demonstrated that service-learning can facilitate occupational therapy students' abilities to be flexible, to be collaborative, and to reflect on the ambiguities of working with others in community (Flecky & Gitlow, 2006; Gitlow & Flecky, 2005). These abilities will be needed by healthcare professionals in the healthcare environment of the future.

Although there are a variety of definitions of *service-learning*, its essence is based on a philosophy of learning by doing in collaborative relationship with community. An overview of major universities, college Web sites, and informational brochures points to the rapid growth of service-learning initiatives within the past decade. Service-learning is a form of community engagement and experiential education that ultimately has a vision or educational paradigm of learning as a means of fostering democratic principles and social change. It engages students, faculty, staff, and community alike in the process of breaking down the barriers that separate campus from community by working with community agencies, organizations, or groups to collectively address community assets and needs to solve community-based concerns. Bringle and Hatcher (1996) stated, "We view service-learning as a credit-bearing educational experience in which students participate in an organized service activity that meets identified community needs and reflect on the service activity in such a way as to gain further understanding of course content, a broader appreciation of the discipline, and an enhanced sense of civic responsibility" (p. 221).

Furthermore, occupational therapy professional education through use of service-learning experiences can foster professional occupational therapy students who exemplify "habits of the heart," or genuine compassion, care and shared vision of a greater community and notion of American society through community partnerships (Bellah, Madson, Sullivan, & Swidler, 1985). The chapters in this book represent a commitment to a shared vision of occupational therapy education that promotes student habits of the heart as well as the knowledge and skills to engage in collaborative dialogue and relationships across diverse groups and communities. In a time of economic uncertainty and cynicism, the habits of genuine, heartfelt interpersonal communication and partnership can promote a community that is hopeful and looks forward to the future together (Arnett & Arneson, 1999).

OVERVIEW OF CONTENTS

Service-Learning in Occupational Therapy Education: Philosophy and Practice is a unique collaboration of insights from occupational therapy educators. They share their expertise on use of service-learning to align occupational therapy education to the future of practice, which meets not only individual occupational needs, but societal and community needs as well.

Chapters 1 and 2 provide an introduction that situates service-learning within the contexts of higher education and occupational therapy philosophy, education, and practice as a way to frame service-learning pedagogy. Chapter 1 details the foundations of service-learning through review of service-learning definitions and use in higher education, and, specifically, occupational therapy education. Chapter 2 describes how to prepare students for future practice using philosophical and theoretical principles of service-learning in relationship to occupational therapy philosophical and pedagogical traditions.

An important goal of this book is to illuminate service-learning through practical examples of how different institutions and occupational therapy program partnerships have met success and challenges in crafting service-learning courses. Chapters 3 through 10 describe effective service-learning partnerships and educational strategies in the community through case studies of service-learning in occupational therapy programs across the United States. Examples of how to design, implement, and assess service-learning projects and partnerships are described along with insights and lessons learned from faculty engaging in service-learning.

Samples of syllabi, readings, Web sites, assignments, and assessments are provided to link service-learning specifically to occupational therapy education and to encourage faculty to explore service-learning for course and curricular use. Important contributions to service-learning theory and research are illustrated in "lessons learned" from faculty, including the strengths and challenges of service-learning based on qualitative and quantitative assessment results and community-based research. Examples of community partnerships, course objectives, and syllabi aligned with Accreditation Council of Occupational Therapy Education (ACOTE) guidelines, readings, Web sites, and course support materials, as well as project and student assessment tools, are provided to illustrate relevant use of service-learning in a variety of occupational therapy coursework.

The book concludes with Chapter 11, which provides a commentary of service-learning in the context of professional formation and fieldwork, and Chapter 12, a summary of service-learning in occupational therapy education with a look to the future of professional education. Although service-learning is apparent in occupational therapy education, we have much to learn about its use and the use of other pedagogical strategies to enhance the professional formation and core competencies and skills of occupational therapy professionals. This is not the start or end of occupational therapy educator collaboration, but a continuing conversation of questioning and promoting best practice in occupational therapy education.

REFERENCES

Arnett, R. C., & Arneson, P. (1999). *Dialogic civility in a cynical age: Community, hope and interpersonal relationships.* Albany, NY: SUNY Press.

Bellah, R., Madson, W. M., Sullivan, A., & Swidler, S. M. (1985). *Habits of the heart: Individualism and commitment in American society.* Berkeley: University of California Press.

Bringle, R .G., & Hatcher, J. A. (1996). Implementing service-learning in higher education. *Journal of Higher Education, 67*(2), 221–239.

Flecky, K., & Gitlow, L. (2006, April). Preparing students for messy practice: Critical reasoning and reflection through service-learning. American Occupational Therapy Association Annual Meeting, Charlotte, NC.

Gitlow, L., & Flecky, K. (2002, May). Service-learning: An action plan for OT educators for the twenty-first century. American Occupational Therapy Association Annual Meeting, Miami, FL.

Gitlow, L., & Flecky, K. (2005). Integrating disability studies concepts into occupational therapy education using service learning. *American Journal of Occupational Therapy, 59,* 546–553.

Acknowledgments

We gratefully dedicate this book and acknowledge the following groups and individuals who contributed to making the dream of this book a reality:

Occupational therapy students and community partners from Husson University and Creighton University who inspire us to become better teachers, collaborators, and citizens. In particular we would like to thank Architect Denis Pratt, AlphaOne, VSA Arts of Maine as well as Blackburn High School, Omaha Street School, Sacred Heart Ministries, and HELP Adult Services in Omaha, Nebraska, for their ongoing collaboration.

Occupational therapy educators who have graciously shared course materials and service-learning experiences with us in order to enhance occupational therapy education.

Family and friends for their support and love.

Christopher Bates and Robert Churchill for their editing guidance and skills.

Kristine Jones and Maro Gartside from Jones and Bartlett for their positive attitude, continuing guidance, and support throughout this book project.

Contributing Authors

Karen Atler, MS, OTR/L
Assistant Professor
Occupational Therapy Department
Colorado State University

Patricia Crist, PhD, OTR, FAOTA
Founding Chair and Professor
Department of Occupational Therapy
Program Director
PhD Program in Rehabilitation Science
Duquesne University

Doris T. Davis
Director
Tillery People's Clinic
Area Wide Health Committee
Concerned Citizens of Tillery

Joy D. Doll, OTD, OTR/L
Assistant Professor
Department of Occupational Therapy
School of Pharmacy and Health Professions
Core Faculty
Office of Interprofessional Scholarship, Service, and Education (OISSE)
Creighton University

Gary R. Grant
Executive Director
Concerned Citizens of Tillery

Kristin Haas, OTD, OTR/L
Assistant Professor
Department of Occupational Therapy
College of St. Mary

Anne Marie Witchger Hansen, MS, OTR/L
Instructor
Department of Occupational Therapy
Rangos School of Health Sciences
Duquesne University

Kimberly Hartmann, PhD, OTR/L, FAOTA
Associate Professor
Chairperson of Occupational Therapy
Department of Occupational Therapy
Quinnipiac University

Roger I. Ideishi, JD, OT/L
Associate Professor
Department of Occupational Therapy
University of the Sciences in Philadelphia

Jaime Phillip Muñoz, PhD, OTR, FAOTA
Associate Professor
Department of Occupational Therapy
Rangos School of Health Sciences
Duquesne University

Ingrid M. Provident, EdD, OTR/L
Assistant Professor and Academic Fieldwork Coordinator
Department of Occupational Therapy
Rangos School of Health Sciences
Duquesne University

Diane Sauter-Davis, MA, OTR/L
Occupational Therapy Assistant Program Director
Kennebec Valley Community College

Beth P. Velde, PhD, OTR/L
Assistant Dean
College of Allied Health Sciences
Professor
Occupational Therapy Department
East Carolina University

Callie Watson, OTD, OTR/L
Associate Professor
Program Director
College of St. Mary

Reviewers

Timothy L. Blasius, EdD, MOT, OTR, LMSW
Assistant Professor
Occupational Therapy Department
Saginaw Valley State University

Elizabeth A. Cada, EdD, OTR/L, FAOTA
Chair
Occupational Therapy Department
College of Health and Human Services
Governors State University

Cathy Dawson, MPA, OTR/L
Assistant Professor
Occupational Therapy
Tuskegee University

John D. Fleming, MOT, OTR/L
Assistant Professor
Occupational Science and Occupational Therapy Department
College of Saint Catherine

Gwendolyn Gray, PhD, OTR/L
Assistant Professor and Director
Occupational Therapy Program
Tuskegee University

Theresa A. Vallone, MS, OTR
Assistant Professor
Academic Fieldwork Coordinator
Occupational Therapy
D'Youville College

Kristin Ann Winston, PhD, OTR/L
Assistant Professor
Master of Occupational Therapy Program
University of Southern Maine

Chapter 1

Foundations of Service-Learning

Kathleen Flecky, OTD, OTR/L

This chapter offers foundational knowledge of service-learning by providing an overview of the discipline's key concepts and definitions. It also features a discussion of relevant theoretical and pedagogical approaches to service-learning and a brief history of service-learning in the United States. Service-learning's relevance in higher education, in general, and education in the health sciences and occupational therapy, in particular, is also explored. Finally, the chapter includes critiques of service-learning as well as a brief summary of trends for service-learning in higher education.

DEFINITIONS OF SERVICE-LEARNING

What is service-learning? Although there are a variety of definitions, the essence of service-learning rests on a philosophy of service and learning that occurs in experiences, reflection, and civic engagement within a collaborative relationship involving community partners. A unique aspect of service-learning is that it incorporates structured opportunities for students, faculty, and community partners to reflect on their interactions and activities in light of both educational and community objectives. The hyphen between *service* and *learning* is purposeful; it denotes a balance between the service and learning outcomes resulting from the partnership experience.

As stated by Jacoby (1996), "Service-learning is a form of experiential education in which students engage in activities that address human and community needs together with structured opportunities intentionally designed to promote student learning and development" (p. 5). This definition differentiates service-learning from other forms of active learning, such as collaborative, cooperative, and problem-based education. Service-learning engages faculty and students with community partners in structured opportunities to meet academic learning objectives while addressing acknowledged community needs. Service-learning is different from volunteer experiences because of the explicit link of course objectives with structured community interactions to meet community-driven needs. Additionally, civic engagement and reflection about service are essential elements of service-learning, which often distinguishes it from internships (Howard, 2001).

According to Eyler & Giles (1999), quality service-learning experiences include the following components: curricula and projects that are sustainable and developed in partnership with the community; activities that are meaningful to student learning and community needs; a clear and relevant connection of community activities to course learning objectives; and purposeful challenges for participants to grapple with diversity and social issues. Service-learning is characterized as the interplay of service and learning, not only within individual course settings, but also within the broader academic institutional goals of community engagement. Brown (2001) describes service-learning as ". . . expanding educational institutions' (and the individual representatives of those institutions) participation *in* community, especially in terms of fostering coalitions and creating responsive resources for and with that community . . ." (p. 5).

The conceptual foundation of occupation and occupational therapy is an ongoing discussion and conversation featuring multiple interdisciplinary theories and applied reference models (Kielhofner, 2004; Kramer, Hinojosa, & Royeen, 2003). Similar to the concept of occupation, service-learning is complex and based on diverse theoretical constructs, which will be described in the next section. As service-learning continues to expand into more courses, curricular models, and institutional infrastructures, theoretical concepts and definitions of service-learning will likely be further delineated and refined to meet the civic and social missions of institutions (Maurrasse, 2004; Shumer & Shumer, 2005).

THEORETICAL AND PEDAGOGICAL APPROACHES

As noted by Howard (1998), ". . . academic service learning is a pedagogical model that intentionally integrates academic service learning and relevant community service" (p. 22). Service-learning is not simply the addition of a service assignment to a course, rather it challenges the teacher, learner, and community partners to connect course materials explicitly to service in community with others, thereby necessitating communal and reciprocal theoretical and pedagogical approaches.

Early writings and research on service-learning frequently cite the work of philosopher John Dewey as the philosophical and pedagogical inspiration for experiential, democratic, and civic education and for service-learning (Giles & Eyler, 1994; Stanton, Giles, & Cruz, 1999). Dewey, a naturalistic philosopher, believed that we reflect and use prior knowledge from experiences to further our growth. The influences of Dewey's works on philosophy and epistemology lead to new ways of thinking about education as actively connecting knowledge to experience through engagement in and reflection on the world outside the classroom (Noddings, 1998). Dewey also linked the purpose of education to promoting democratic instructional practices and a more fully democratic society (Dewey, 1916). Dewey wrote:

> A society which makes provisions for participation in its good of all members on equal terms and which secures flexible readjustment of its institutions through interaction of the different forms of associated life is in so far democratic. Such a society must have a type of education which gives individuals

a personal interest in social relationships and control, and the habits of mind which secure social changes without introducing disorder. (p. 99)

In addition to Dewey, the theoretical insights of David Kolb and Donald Schon on the role of reflective thinking in experiential education have influenced how pedagogy incorporates reflection on service as integral to service-learning (Cone & Harris, 1996; Eyler, Giles, & Schmiede, 1996). Kolb's cycle process (Kolb, 1984)—reflection on concrete experiences, thoughtful observation, abstract conceptualization, and active experimentation—lead to inclusion of reflective activities prior to, during, and after service as part of service-learning assignments. Schon's practice of reflection in action and his reciprocal reflection teaching and coaching model (Schon, 1987) have been used to foster reciprocal reflective activities among students, faculty, and community partners (Honnet & Poulsen, 1989).

Service-learning also draws on critical theory and feminist pedagogy (Brown, 2001; Deans, 1999). As noted by Friere (1973) and Shor (1987), critical theory emphasizes that education is political and should involve a dialectical approach of problem-posing and a critique of social systems and the civic responsibilities of education. Feminist pedagogy also espouses the need for critical reflection and dialogue related to educational aspects of privilege and power (Weiler, 1991). These models point to the importance of situating service-learning in context with social issues and challenges. The development of participatory-action and community-based research in service-learning are examples of how these pedagogies support community advocacy and give greater voice to community partners with their strengths and needs (Strand, Marullo, Cutforth, Stoecker, & Donohue, 2003; Reardon, 1998).

Finally, in addition to the use of social learning and cognitive learning models, recent development in service-learning theoretical frameworks include the use of a pedagogy of engagement (Lowery et al., 2006), the transformational model (Kiely, 2005), and service-learning as postmodern pedagogy (Butin, 2005). Each of these models has promise in helping to elucidate service-learning as a concept of teaching and learning with important philosophical considerations based on current research. As the theory of service-learning is more fully developed, researchers can apply theory to gain a clearer understanding of the impact and value of service-learning as a philosophy and pedagogy.

In summary, the diversity of theoretical and pedagogical approaches described in this section can be viewed as both a concern and as strength. Numerous sources point to an urgent need for a logical and relevant theoretical basis for service-learning and note the concerns of multiple, diverse theories to support needed evidence-based research studies (Langana & Rubin, 2001; Billig & Welch, 2004). However, some authors have posited that service-learning is a complex philosophical and pedagogical concept, one best served by multiple models of origin and through research, pedagogical discussion, and the critique of a variety of theoretical models (Butin, 2005). Clearly, it is important that educators, students, community partners, and institutions understand the history of service-learning before incorporating service-learning into courses or curricula.

THE HISTORY OF SERVICE-LEARNING IN HIGHER EDUCATION

Many universities and colleges were founded to serve their communities as well as educate their citizens. Service-learning's philosophical roots lie in social-reform movements, as exemplified by Jane Addams and Hull House in the late 1800s, and the educational reform movements of Dewey and others at the University of Chicago in the early 1900s (Titlebaum, Williamson, Daprano, Baer, & Brahler, 2004). Schools of higher learning, especially the land-grant colleges in the 1900s, developed extension programs that initially focused on the needs of the local farming communities and the Work Projects Administration during the Great Depression (Kenny & Gallagher, 2002).

After World War II, the federal government, through the G.I. Bill, partnered with higher education to provide funding and opportunities for former servicemen to obtain college degrees. Higher education became more readily available to the middle class, which resulted in members of many different communities sharing their educational skills with others. Furthermore, in the 1940s and 1950s many universities and colleges continued to meet communities' needs regionally and locally through cooperative-education programs and student volunteer experiences. The emergence of the Civil Rights Movement, the Peace Corps, and VISTA (Volunteers in Service to America) programs in the 1960s, sparked a resurgence in the growth of national civic responsibility and community service on college campuses well into the 1980s and 1990s (National Service-Learning Clearinghouse, 2008).

Following the establishment the Campus Outreach Opportunity League in 1984 and The National Campus Compact (a coalition of university and college presidents) in 1985, additional organizations began to link the mission of universities and colleges and students across the United States with the promotion of civic responsibility and engagement through service (National Service-Learning Clearinghouse, 2008).

The 1990s featured continuing growth of campus service organizations with an expanding educational movement to link academic institutions to communities through teaching, research, and service. Ernest Boyer (1996), a leader in higher education, asserted that the role of institutions and faculty of higher education should be to support communities through engagement in the application of knowledge, as well as the discovery and integration of knowledge, through working with communities in needed community-based research, teaching, and service.

The National and Community Service Act of 1990 and the establishment of the Learn and Serve America Corps, along with Campus Compact, created a national structure to support academic–community initiatives (Titlebaum, Williamson, Daprano, Baer, & Brahler, 2004). The growth of these national organizations supported Boyer's notion of educational institutions in partnership with communities and the scholarship of engagement as relevant to current initiatives in community service (Boyer, 1996). Service-learning initiatives that began in the early 1980s became the early precursors to the phenomenal growth of service-learning programs across the United States in 1990s. Based on a 2007 member survey, Campus Compact reported more than 950 institutions and affiliated state offices in more than 30 states (Campus Compact, 2008).

Today, many academic–community partnerships are visible through service-learning and civic-engagement activities on many U.S. campuses. Campus Compact (2008) reports the following on its member institutions: "... On average, campuses have 77 community partnerships each, involving a range of nonprofit/community-based organizations, K-12 schools, faith-based organizations, and government agencies ..." (p. 2).

With a similar growth of service-learning in K-12 learning communities (Root, Callahan, & Billig, 2005), many students entering colleges and universities will already have experience with service-learning. Therefore, students are increasingly viewed as partners and leaders in service-learning programs on college campuses (Zlotkowski, Longo, & Williams, 2007). As student, faculty, institutional, and community partnerships continue to flourish and become integrated with campus infrastructures, there is growing call for rigorous research and analysis of the impact of service-learning as practiced in higher education.

SERVICE-LEARNING RESEARCH IN HIGHER EDUCATION

Although the research on service-learning has been questioned in terms of its methodology and rigor, studies indicate that service-learning has a positive impact on students' attitudes toward community engagement and citizenship, as well as their growth in interpersonal activities, civic responsibility, and problem-solving skills (Eyler & Giles, 1999; Eyler, Giles, Stentson, & Gray, 2001; Moely, McFarland, Miron, Mercer, & Ilustre, 2002). Much of the initial research on service-learning centered on positive student learning outcomes and the impact of service participation on students' attitudes, values, and beliefs (Astin & Sax, 1998; Markus, Howard, & King, 1993). Additional studies and literature have investigated how best to improve service-learning programming, assessment, and institutional culture for positive academic and community outcomes (Furco, 2002; Gelmon, Holland, Driscoll, Spring, & Kerrigan, 2001; Schneider, 1998). Recent studies have addressed the impact of service-learning on how community partners view student–faculty–institutional interactions and contributions to the community. Community partners appreciate their role as student educators and the resources academic members bring to their settings (Sandy & Holland, 2006; Worrall, 2007).

Literature on education and the community has addressed the value of community partnership relationships and enhancing community benefits in service-learning, best practices for service-learning programming, and emerging international service-learning, as noted in the *Michigan Journal of Community Service Learning,* the *Journal of Higher Education, Educational Leadership,* and *Teaching and Teacher Education.* Just as studies have demonstrated the value of service-learning, limitations of these studies and criticisms of service-learning pedagogy have emerged.

Limitations and critiques of service-learning involve consideration of some student experiences that actually reinforce stereotypes or that reflect the volunteer or charity model of "doing for" instead of a collaborative partnership of "doing with" the community (Brown, 2001; Egger, 2007). Theoretical foundations of service-learning have also been criticized as lacking substance and clear conceptualization (Butin, 2006; Sheffield, 2005). Recent literature in service-learning in K-12 and higher education has reinforced the call for a theoretical framework of service-learning as well as key concepts/components of service-learning based on theory (Root, Callahan, & Billig, 2005). Although studies indicate positive benefits of service-learning, the robustness of research has been questioned with a renewed call for more rigorous and sophisticated research designs and examination of longitudinal impacts of service-learning on students, faculty members, community partners, academic institutions, and the community (Eyler, 2002).

A current initiative within higher education is to investigate the role of the scholarship of engagement and research within institutions. In a recent conference report, "New Times Demand New Scholarship II: Research Universities and Civic Engagement—Opportunities and Challenges," the authors recommended that ". . . our zeal for engaging students in service-learning and community-based research should be matched by scholarly efforts to understand and articulate systematically the outcomes, challenges, and best practices in this work. Such inquiry should be undertaken at the course level, as well as across disciplines, schools, and institutions" (Stanton, 2007, p. 13). A systematic, institution-wide appraisal of the use of service-learning and community engagement may lead to more intentional research on theory and the application of service-learning.

SERVICE-LEARNING IN THE HEALTH SCIENCES

Integrating professional healthcare education with engagement in the community is becoming increasingly common across disciplines in the health sciences. Literature from the fields of medicine, nursing, occupational therapy, physical therapy, public health, social work, and others indicates both benefits and challenges of incorporating service-learning as part of their curricula and as interdisciplinary experiences (Hodges & Videto, 2008; Gitlow & Flecky, 2005; Gutheil, Cheraesky, & Sherratt, 2006; Kearney, 2008; Peabody, Block, & Jain, 2008). Students benefit from opportunities to develop knowledge and skills working with faculty and community partners in real-life situations and settings, and communities benefit from joint partnerships that provide health-related services and resources (Brush, Markert, & Lazarus, 2006; Dorfman, Murty, Ingram, & Li, 2007; Lashley, 2007).

As healthcare trends indicate the movement of service-delivery into more outpatient and community settings, with an emphasis on preventative care and health promotion, health professional students will benefit from opportunities to interact and engage with individuals and agencies in the community setting (Gregorio, DeChello, & Segal, 2008; Institute of Medicine, 2007). Additionally, service-learning provides an opportunity for schools of health to fulfill their mission of addressing health disparities and community health needs while meeting education standards set by national accreditation bodies.

Challenges of service-learning for the health sciences are similar to those experienced by faculty, students, and community partners in higher education. These may include lack of knowledge or resources to incorporate service-learning in existing courses or to create new coursework; resistance to service-learning; or logistical difficulties in terms of community scheduling; lack of time needed for communication, collaboration, and planning; and limited funding for programming (Holland, 1999). Although research shows that faculty are frequently the leaders in promoting service-learning on campus, some faculty may be hesitant to incorporate or sustain service-learning in their courses because of barriers such as those previously noted or because of pressures to meet institutional promotion and tenure guidelines (Sandmann, Foster-Fishman, Lloyd, Rauhe, & Rosaen, 2000; Abes, Jackson, & Jones, 2002).

Some institutions of higher education are incorporating the scholarship of engagement as characterized by Boyer (1996) as important aspects of faculty work in the areas of research, teaching, and scholarship. Recently, The Carnegie Foundation has established a community-engagement institutional classification, which provides national recognition for the unique strategies that institutions promote and demonstrate to enhance community engagement (Driscoll, 2008). This classification may provide faculty and institutional members with renewed energy and recognition for making service-learning and community engagement visible and sustainable.

SERVICE-LEARNING IN OCCUPATIONAL THERAPY

How is service-learning exemplified in occupational therapy education? As will be discussed throughout this text in contributor chapters, service-learning provides a contextually relevant and rich educational environment for students to actively apply occupation-based theories and skills to real-world occupational performance needs that are identified as important by a particular community. Nationally and internationally, a review of the literature in occupational-therapy-related journals shows an increase of publications on service-learning in occupational therapy and interdisciplinary health programs (Alsop, 2007; Beck & Barnes, 2007; Gitlow & Flecky, 2005; Hoppes, Bender, & DeGrace, 2005; Lohman & Aitken, 2002; Lorenzo,

Duncan, Bachanan, & Alsop, 2006; O'Brien & D'Amico, 2004; Waskiewicz, 2002; Witchger-Hansen et al. 2007).

In recent years, community engagement and service-learning topics have been featured in numerous presentations at the American Occupational Therapy Association (American Occupational Therapy Association [AOTA], 2008; 2007; 2006; 2005; 2004; 2003). Service-learning coalition consortia have also emerged across the United States and abroad that include occupational therapy faculty and students (Campus Compact, 2008; Center for Healthy Communities, 2007: Community-Campus Partnerships for Health, n.d.; Midwest Consortium of Service-Learning in Higher Education, n.d.).

Service-learning, as a form of community engagement, has been used as a relevant teaching and learning tool in a variety of courses and student experiences, as evidenced in the chapters in this text. We encourage you to explore the various types of community partnerships, student and faculty experiences, reflective strategies, assessment and outcome tools, and lessons learned in the chapters that follow.

FINAL THOUGHTS

Butin (2005) states that service-learning can be dangerous when used as an educational pedagogy and theoretical framework. It is dangerous in that it calls into question the traditional notion that education is separated from the larger community. It asks educators to view learning as an act of challenging students to become better citizens and demonstrate the ideals of democracy and social justice. It calls on us to blur the roles of student-educator and community and share power, expertise, and resources for a common mission and vision of community. The community is viewed as a partner and a collaborator rather than as a vague entity that students come from and graduate into. It is dangerous because it is a powerful way to mentor students to share their knowledge and skills for others rather than to settle for students who demonstrate knowledge and skills but lack the resources to move into future areas of practice.

One of the core values and beliefs of the occupational therapy profession is that "dignity emphasizes the importance of valuing the inherent worth and uniqueness of each person. This value is demonstrated by an attitude of empathy and respect for self and other" (American Occupational Therapy Association, 1993, p. 1085). In the occupational therapy service-learning courses I have engaged in with students and community partners over the years, we have experienced three moments of learning about human dignity: (1) the realization noted by students that they "serve" in many ways—most importantly as a catalyst and a witness to empowering others to serve themselves; (2) the process of service, an interdependence and shared vulnerability, emerges as students view themselves as change agents for others; and (3) the inherent humanness of us all—we all have limitations, and, in fact, our limitations present an opportunity for strength in collaboration. Limitations and strengths come in many forms—financial, political, physical, social, cultural—and student insight from analysis of these strengths and limitations of themselves and others fuels a developmental process of becoming a change agent.

Service-learning provides a potent tool for service and learning. How do we choose to dignify our profession of occupational therapy? Perhaps by educating future occupational therapy professionals in ways that reframe how we view the community—not as a setting in which we do occupation-based intervention, but as a place where we partner with others to create a healthier, more rich way of life. We dignify clients when we care about where they come from and where they are going. Community is more than an intervention setting—it is where we live and relate with others *in community*. It is dangerous thinking.

REFERENCES

Abes, E. S., Jackson, G., & Jones, S. R. (2002). Factors that motivate and deter faculty use of service-learning. *Michigan Journal of Community Service Learning, 9*(1), 5–17.

Alsop, A. (2007). Service-learning: The challenge of civic responsibility. *British Journal of Occupational Therapy, 70*(4), 139.

American Occupational Therapy Association. (1993). Core values and attitudes of occupational therapy practice. *American Journal of Occupational Therapy, 47,* 1085–1086.

American Occupational Therapy Association (2008). *The American Occupational Therapy Association's 88th Annual Conference & Expo Conference Program Guide.* Bethesda, MD: Author.

American Occupational Therapy Association. (2007). *The American Occupational Therapy Association's 87th Annual Conference & Expo Conference Program Guide.* Bethesda, MD: Author.

American Occupational Therapy Association. (2006). *The American Occupational Therapy Association's 86th Annual Conference & Expo Conference Program Guide.* Bethesda, MD: Author.

American Occupational Therapy Association. (2005). *The American Occupational Therapy Association's 85th Annual Conference & Expo Conference Program Guide.* Bethesda, MD: Author.

American Occupational Therapy Association. (2004). *The American Occupational Therapy Association's 84th Annual Conference & Expo Conference Program Guide.* Bethesda, MD: Author.

American Occupational Therapy Association. (2003). *The American Occupational Therapy Association's 83th Annual Conference & Expo Conference Program Guide.* Bethesda, MD: Author.

Astin, A. W., & Sax, L. (1998). How undergraduates are affected by service participation. *Journal of College Student Development, 39*(3), 251–263.

Beck, A. J., Barnes, K. J. (2007). Reciprocal service-learning: Texas border Head Start and Master of occupational therapy students. *Occupational Therapy in Health Care, 21*(1/2), 7–23.

Billig, S. H., & Welch, M. (2004). Service-learning as civically engaged scholarship: Challenges and strategies in higher education and K–12 settings. In M. Welch & S.H. Billig (Eds.), *New perspectives in service-learning: Research to advance the field* (pp. 221–242). Greenwich, CT: Information Age Publishing.

Boyer, E. (1996). The scholarship of engagement. *Journal of Public Outreach, 1*(1), 11–20.

Brown, D. (2001). *Pulling it together: A method for developing service-learning and community partnerships based on critical pedagogy.* Washington, DC: Corporation for National Service.

Brush, D. R., Markert, R. J., & Lazarus, C. J. (2006). The relationship between service learning and medical student academic and professional outcomes. *Teaching and Learning in Medicine, 18*(1), 9–13.

Butin, D. W. (2005). Service-learning as postmodern pedagogy. In *Service-learning in higher education* (pp. 89–104). New York: Palgrave Macmillan.

Butin, D. W. (2006). The limits of service-learning in higher education. *The Review of Higher Education, 29*(4), 473–498.

Campus Compact. (2008). *2007 Service Statistics: Highlights and Trends of Campus Compact's Annual Membership Survey.* Providence, RI: Campus Compact.

Center for Healthy Communities. (2007). Midwest Health Professions Service Learning Consortium. Retrieved December 5, 2008, from http://www.med.wright.edu/chc.tech/techsl.htm.

Community-Campus Partnerships for Health. (n.d.). Community-Campus partnerships for health: Transforming communities & higher education. Retrieved October 10, 2008, from http://depts.washington.edu/ccph/guide.html.

Cone, D., & Harris, S. (1996). Service learning practice: Developing a theoretical framework. *Michigan Journal of Community Service Learning, 3*(Fall), 31–43.

Deans, T. (1999). Service-learning in two keys: Paulo Freire's critical pedagogy in relation to John Dewey's pragmatism. *Michigan Journal of Community Service Learning, 6,* 5–29.

Dewey, J. (1916). *Democracy and education: An introduction to the philosophy of education.* New York: The Free Press.

Dorfman, L. T., Murty, S. A., Ingram, J. G., & Li, H. (2007). Evaluating the outcomes of gerontological curriculum enrichment: A multi-modal approach. *Gerontology & Geriatrics Education, 27*(4), 1–21.

Driscoll, A. (2008). Carnegie's community engagement classification: Intentions and insights. *Change,* January–February, 39–41.

Egger, J. B. (2007). Service 'learning' reduces learning. *The Examiner.* Retrieved December 21, 2007, from http://www.examiner.com/a-966679˜John_B__Egger__Service__lea rning__reduces_learning.html.

Eyler, J., & Giles, D. E. Jr. (1999). *Where's the learning in service-learning?* San Francisco: Jossey-Bass.

Eyler, J., Giles, D. E. Jr., & Schmiede, A. (1996). *A practitioner's guide to reflection in service-learning: Student voices & reflections.* Nashville, TN: Vanderbilt University.

Eyler, J., Giles, D. E. Jr., Stentson, C. M., & Gray, C. J. (2001). *At a glance: What we know about the effects of service-learning on college students, faculty, institutions and communities, 1993–2000.* (3rd ed.). Nashville, TN: Vanderbilt University.

Eyler, J. (2002). Stretching to meet the challenge: Improving the quality of research to improve the quality of service-learning. In S. H. Billing & A. Furco (Eds.), *Service-learning through a multidisciplinary lens* (pp. 3–13). Greenwich, CT: Information Age Publishing.

Freire, P. (1973). *Education for critical consciousness.* New York: Continuum Publishing.

Furco, A. (2002). Institutionalizing service-learning in higher education. *Journal of Public Affairs, 6*(Suppl. 1), 39–67.

Gelmon, S. B., Holland, B. A., Driscoll, A., Spring, A., & Kerrigan, S. (2001). *Assessing service-learning and civic engagement: Principles and techniques.* Providence, RI: Compass Compact.

Giles, D. E. Jr., & Eyler, J. (1994). Theoretical roots of service learning in John Dewey: Toward a theory of service learning. *Michigan Journal of Community Service Learning,* Fall, 77–85.

Gitlow, L., & Flecky, K. (2005). Integrating disability studies concepts into occupational therapy education using service learning. *American Journal of Occupational Therapy, 59,* 546–553.

Gregorio, D. I., DeChello, L. M., & Segal, J. (2008). *Public Health, 123*(Suppl. 2), 44–52.

Gutheil, I. A., Cheraesky, R. H., & Sherratt, M. L. (2006). *Educational Gerontology, 32*(9), 771–784.

Hodges, B. C., & Videto, D. M. (2008). *American Journal of Health Education, 39*(1), 44–54.

Holland, B. (1999). Factors and strategies that influence faculty involvement in public service. *Journal of Public Service and Outreach, 4*(1), 37–43.

Honnet, E. P., & Poulsen, S. (1989). *Principles of good practice in combining service and learning: Wingspread special report.* Racine, WI: Johnson Foundation.

Hoppes, S., Bender, D., DeGrace, B. W. (2005). *Journal of Allied Health, 34*(1), 47–50.

Howard, J. P. E. (1998). Academic service learning: A counternormative pedagogy. *New Directions for Teaching and Learning, 73,* 21–29.

Howard, J. (2001). *Michigan Journal of Community Service-Learning: Service-learning course design workbook.* Ann Arbor, MI: OCSL Press.

Institute of Medicine (2007). *Retooling for an Aging America; Building the HealthCare Workforce.* Washington, DC: National Academies Press.

Jacoby, B., & Associates (Eds.). (1996). *Service-learning in higher education: Concepts and practices.* San Francisco: Jossey-Bass.

Jenkins, G., Douglas, F., & Chamberlain, E. (2008). Compulsory volunteering: Using service-learning to introduce occupation to occupational therapy students. *British Journal of Occupational Therapy, 71*(1), 38–40.

Kearney, K. R. (2008). A service-learning course for first-year pharmacy students. *American Journal of Pharmacy Education, 72*(4), 86.

Kenny, M. E., & Gallagher, L. A. (2002). Service-learning: A history of systems. In M. E. Kenny, L. A. Simon, K. Kiley-Bradeck, & R. M. Lerner (Eds.), *Learning to serve: Promoting civil society through service learning* (pp. 15–29). Boston: Kluwer Publishers.

Keilhofner, G. (2004). *Conceptual Foundations of Occupational Therapy.* Philadelphia, PA; F.A. Davis Co.

Kiely, R. (2005). A transformative learning model for service-learning: a longitudinal case study. *Michigan Journal of Community Service Learning, (12),* 5–22.

Kolb, D. A. (1984). *Experiential learning: Experience as the source of learning and development.* Englewood Cliffs, NJ: Prentice Hall.

Kramer, P., Hinojosa, J. & Royeen, C. B. (Ed.). (2003). *Perspectives on Human Occupation: Participation in Life.* Philadelphia: Lippincott, Williams & Wilkins.

Langana, L., & Rubin, M. S. (2001). Methodological challenges and potential solutions for the incorporation of sound community-based research into service-learning. In A. Furco & S. H. Billig (Eds.), *Service-learning: The essence of the pedagogy* (pp. 161–182). Greenwich, CT: Information Age Publishing.

Lashley, M. (2007). Nurses on a mission: A professional service learning experience with the inner city homeless. *Nursing Education Perspectives, 28*(1), 24–26.

Lohman, H., & Aitken, M. J. (2002). Occupational therapy students' attitudes toward service learning. *Physical and Occupational Therapy in Geriatrics, 20*(3–4), 155–164.

Lorenzo, T., Duncan, M., Buchanan, H., & Alsop, A. (Eds.). (2006). *Practice and service learning in occupational therapy: Enhancing potential in context.* West Sussex, England: Whurr.

Lowery, D., May, D. L., Duchane, K. A., Coulter-Kern, R., Bryant, D., Morris, P. V., et al. (2006). A logic model of service-learning: tensions and issues for further consideration. *Michigan Journal of Community Service Learning, 12,* 47–60.

Markus, G. B., Howard, J., & King, D. (1993). Integrating community service and classroom instruction enhances learning: Results from an experiment. *Educational Evaluation and Policy Analysis, 15*(4), 410–419.

Maurrasse, D. (2004). Leadership, strategy, and change: Challenges in forging timely and effective learning communities. In J. A. Galura, P. A. Pasque, D. Schoem, & J. Howard (Eds.), *Engaging the whole of service-learning, diversity, and learning opportunities* (pp. 8–13). Ann Arbor: OCSL Press at the University of Michigan.

Midwest Consortium for Service-Learning in Higher Education. (n.d.). Welcome to the Midwest Consortium for Service-learning in Higher Education. Retrieved January 2, 2009, from http://themidwestconsortium.googlepages.com/.

Moely, B. E., McFarland, M., Miron, D., Mercer, S., & Ilustre, V. (2002). Changes in college students' attitudes and intentions for civic involvement as a function of service-learning experiences. *Michigan Journal of Service Learning, 8*(2), 15–26.

National Service-Learning Clearinghouse. (2008). Annotated history of service-learning: 1862–2002. Retrieved October 30, 2008, from http://www.servicelearning.org/filemanager/download/142/SL Comp Timeline 3-15-04_rev.pdf.

Noddings, N. (1998). *Philosophy of education.* Boulder, CO: Westview Press.

O'Brien, S. P., & D'Amico, M. L. (2004). Service-learning is the perfect fit for occupational therapy and physical therapy education. *American Occupational Therapy Association Education Special Interest Section Quarterly, 14*(3), 1–3.

Peabody, C., Block, A., & Jain, S. (2008). *Medical Education, 42*(5), 533–534.

Reardon, K. M. (1998). Participatory action research as service learning. In R. Rhoads & J. Howard (Eds.). *Academic service-learning: A pedagogy of action and reflection* (pp. 57–64). San Francisco: Jossey-Bass.

Root, S., Callahan, J., & Billig, S. H. (Eds.). (2005). Introduction. In *Improving service-learning practice: Research on models to enhance impacts* (pp. ix–xii). Greenwich, CT: Information Age Publishing.

Sandmann, L. R., Foster-Fishman, P.G., Lloyd, J., Rauhe, W., and Rosaen, C. (2000). Managing critical tensions: How to strengthen the scholarship component of outreach. *Change 32*(1), 44–52.

Sandy, M., & Holland, B. (2006). Different worlds and common ground: Community partner perspectives on campus-community partnerships. *Michigan Journal of Community Service Learning, 13*(1), 30–43.

Schneider, M. K. (1998). Models of good practice for service learning programs. What can we learn from 1,000 faculty, 25,000 students, and 27 institutions involved in service? *AAHE Bulletin, 50*(10), 9–12.

Schon, D. A. (Ed.). (1987). *Educating the reflective practitioner: Toward a new design for teaching and learning in the professions.* San Francisco: Jossey-Bass.

Sheffield, E. C. (2005). Service in service-learning education: The need for philosophical understanding. *The High School Journal*, October–November, 46–53.

Shor, I. (Ed.). (1987). *Friere for the classroom: A sourcebook for liberatory teaching.* Portsmouth, NH: Boynton/Cook Publishers.

Shor, I., & Freire, P. (1987). *A pedagogy for liberation: Dialogues on transforming education.* South Hadley, MA: Bergin & Garvey Publishers.

Shumer, R., & Shumer, S. S. (2005). Using principles of research to discover multiple levels of connection and engagement: A civic engagement audit. In S. Root, J. Callahan, & S. H. Billig (Eds.), *Improving service-learning practice: Research on models to enhance impacts* (pp. 167–185). Greenwich, CT: Information Age Publishing.

Stanton, T. (2007). New Times Demand New Scholarship II: Research Universities and Civic Engagement—Opportunities and Challenges, University of California; Los Angeles. Retrieved online October 22, 2009, from http://www.compact.org/wp-content/uploads/initiatives/research_universities/Civic_Engagement.pdf.

Stanton, T. K., Giles, D. E. Jr., and Cruz, N. (1999). *Service-learning: A movement's pioneers reflect on its origins, practice, and future.* San Francisco: Jossey-Bass.

Strand, K., Marullo, S., Cutforth, N., Stoecker, R., & Donohue, P. (2003). Principles of best practice for community-based research. *Michigan Journal of Community Service Learning, 9*(3), 5–15.

Titlebaum, P., Williamson, G., Daprano, C., Baer, J., & Brahler, J. (2004). *Annotated History of Service-Learning.* Dayton, Ohio: University of Dayton.

Waskiewicz, R. (2002). Impact of service-learning on occupational therapy students' awareness and sense of responsibility toward community. In S. H. Billing & A. Furco (Eds.). *Service-learning: Through a multidisciplinary lens* (pp. 123–150). Greenwich, CT: Information Age Publishing.

Witchger Hansen, A. M., Muñoz, J. P., Crist, P. Gupta, J., Ideishi, R., Primeau, L. A., et al. (2007). Service learning: Meaningful, community-centered professional skill development for occupational therapy students. *Occupational Therapy in Health Care, 1–2,* 25–49.

Weiler, K. (1991). Friere and a feminist pedagogy of difference. *Harvard Educational Review, 61,* 449–474.

Worrall, L. (2007). Asking the community: A case study of community partner perspectives. *Michigan Journal of Community Service Learning, 14*(1), 5–17.

Zlotkowski, E. A. (1998). *Successful service-learning programs: New models of excellence in higher education.* Boston: Anker Publishing.

Zlotkowski. E., Longo, N. V., & Williams, J. R. (2007). *Students as colleagues: Expanding the circle of service-learning leadership.* Boston: Campus Compact.

Chapter 2

Occupational Therapy Education: Preparing Students for Future Practice

Lynn Gitlow, PhD, OTR/L, ATP

The Centennial Vision for our profession states, "We envision that occupational therapy is a powerful, widely recognized, science-driven, and evidence-based profession with a globally connected and diverse workforce meeting society's occupational needs (AOTA, 2008a)." The American Occupational Therapy Association's (AOTA) Centennial Vision is both ambitious and practicable. Many feasible methods exist to achieve this vision, and the one discussed in this text relates to educating occupational therapy practitioners. In relation to the Centennial Vision, Florence Clark (2006) states, "A new curriculum responsive to the emerging needs of society must be put in place, but it must be based on our time-honored curriculum and values."

The question of how to make the connection with time-honored values while moving our profession forward to meet twenty-first-century healthcare needs has been discussed at length. This chapter extends that discussion. Paramount in this endeavor is the belief that the educational strategy presented here can help occupational therapy practitioners to advance and deliver on our Centennial Vision. As educators move toward the consideration and application of service-learning as a potent educational strategy, it is customary to contextualize the arena of discussion. Therefore, this chapter will review societal issues, the healthcare environment, and occupational therapy education, all of which require deliberation in order to craft a responsive curriculum. Service-learning will be described as a teaching strategy that espouses the underlying values and philosophy of occupational therapy.

SOCIETAL ISSUES THAT IMPACT THE EDUCATION OF FUTURE PRACTITIONERS

"The crisis of our time reveals the dying of an old structure and way of thinking . . ." (Scharmer, 2007, p. 2). Every day you can open the paper or turn on the computer and read of disparities in wealth, education, health care, and equality that are presenting intolerable situations for many of the world's citizens. Former President Clinton calls on all citizens of the world to "do public good." In his book *Giving* (Clinton, 2007), Clinton cites numerous examples of private citizens doing public actions to ensure that in a world of inequality ongoing work continues to guarantee the rights of every person to participate in meaningful occupations by eliminating poverty and promoting health, equality, education, and other services. Calls echo from venues requesting that citizens help stem the inequities that erode the health of many of our world's citizens. Certainly, those of us who provide healthcare services can do our part to create more holistic interactions.

As president-elect, Barack Obama asked all citizens to consider increasing their service to achieve national goals related to health care, education, the environment, and restoring the status of the United States in the world (Obama, 2007). Engaging students in service, which allows them to help with community problem-solving, has been funded by the federal programs such as Learn and Serve America and federal work-study programs. In addition, President Obama has proposed a tuition-reduction package for service-related occupations. Along with other healthcare programs, occupational therapy participates in educational endeavors that address community-based problems that impact the health of citizens (Community-Campus Partnerships on Health, 2008).

The World Health Organization reminds us that threats to health come from a variety of causes, including war, climate change, and human-caused and natural catastrophes (World Health Report, 2007). As occupational therapists, we understand that health is much more than a medical or biological entity. Consistent with the International Classification of Functioning, Disability and Health (ICF), we view health as a complex interaction of contextually related transactions among a person and his/her environments.

Understandably, the threats to health mentioned earlier are certainly of concern to us as we consider promoting participation in meaningful occupations for our clients. More important, educational programs need to be preparing students who can address these issues. The Occupational Therapy Practice Framework: Domain and Process, 2nd edition (AOTA, 2008b) recognizes the multiple factors that are involved in supporting and maintaining health, including client factors as well as contextual and environmental influences. This document delineates that clients for occupational therapy include persons, organizations, and populations. Educational practices must now prepare students to move beyond seeing the individual as the sole focus of our practice.

PROMOTING OCCUPATIONAL JUSTICE AND COMMUNITY INCLUSION

Being able to participate in meaningful occupations, while promoting the health of multiple constituencies, is at the core of occupational therapy. One AOTA paper describes the critical role that occupational therapy practitioners take in emphasizing participation in meaningful occupations as a means of preventing disease and promoting healthy lifestyles (AOTA, 2008a). When occupational therapy practitioners perform interventions within populations, the goal is to address the health of all people in the community, not just those individuals with the resources to obtain services. Enabling all to participate in meaningful occupation has been termed *occupational justice,* and it is now included in the Occupational Therapy Practice Framework: Domain and Process, 2nd edition (AOTA, 2008b) as one of the possible outcomes of occupational therapy intervention.

Wilcock (2006) has written extensively about occupational justice and has noted how important meeting basic needs are in order for a person to experience occupational well-being or health. Threats to basic needs such as poverty, inequality, lack of health care, and so on are relevant to occupational therapists who encounter people as a result of a population's occupational needs. The notion of *population* is a longstanding consideration for our profession. Grady (1995), in her Eleanor Clark Slagle address, urged occupational therapists to be concerned with community inclusion for all, reminding listeners that occupations occur in communities, not in institutions. Finally, our Code of Ethics states that:

> Members of AOTA are committed to promoting inclusion, diversity, independence, and safety for all recipients in various stages of life, health, and illness and to empower all beneficiaries of occupational therapy. This commitment extends beyond service recipients to include professional colleagues, students, educators, businesses, and the community. (AOTA, 2005, p. 639)

As this book attests, occupational therapy programs are rising to meet this challenge.

INFLUENCES FROM THE HEALTHCARE ENVIRONMENT

Great changes in health care, as well as in the definition of *health* itself, are taking place as demographics change and health care advances move healthcare professionals from a primary focus on curing acute illness toward a broader definition of health that includes sustained care for those who have chronic and lifelong illnesses. For occupational therapists, a return to their philosophical roots of defining *health* from a perspective of participating in meaningful occupation, rather than merely an absence of disease, is both timely and consistent with the evolving healthcare arena.

What is it that makes occupational therapy so relevant, or as Mary Reilly (1962) put it, "one of the great ideas of twentieth century medicine?" The underlying beauty and uniqueness of occupational therapy is that it focuses on "supporting health and participation in life through engagement in occupation" (AOTA, 2008b). Two of the most important underpinnings of occupational therapy are active participation and engagement.

"The occupational therapy profession affirms the right of every individual to access and full participation within society" (AOTA, 2004, p. 668). Although our profession strives to meet this lofty goal, many individuals have not reached this destination.

Education is critical to our future professionals as they train to become a unified workforce capable of championing the occupational needs of diverse societies. In fact, the Accreditation Council for Occupational Therapy Education (ACOTE) standards (ACOTE, 2007) for occupational therapy education state that entry occupational therapy practitioners among other things should be able to:

> **B.6.2.** Discuss the current policy issues and the social, economic, political, geographic, and demographic factors that influence the various contexts for practice of occupational therapy.

> **B.6.3.** Describe the current social, economic, political, geographic, and demographic factors to promote policy development and the provision of occupational therapy services.

> **B.6.4.** Articulate the role and responsibility of the practitioner to address changes in service delivery policies to effect changes in the system and to identify opportunities in emerging practice areas.

> **B.6.5.** Articulate the trends in models of service delivery and their potential effect on the practice of occupational therapy, including, but not limited to, medical, educational, community, and social models.

In the Occupational Therapy Practice Framework: Domain and Process, 2nd edition, occupational therapy embraces a holistic view of health, a view that is consistent with the ICF. The reductionist or traditional medical model would narrowly define *health* as the absence of disease. Health is more than the absence of disease. It is the ability to do. As client-centered practitioners we engage our clients in "doing," and focus this "doing" on their wants and needs. This perspective has been called for in a number of documents, including *Crossing the Quality Chasm: A New Health System for the Twenty-First Century* (Institute of Medicine, 2001), which highlights the change from care focused on acute health to that focused on chronic health, with the client as partner. One of the publication's recommendations is that healthcare providers deliver client-centered care. Healthcare providers are also called upon to provide care that does not vary in quality because of personal characteristics such as gender, ethnicity, geographic location, and socioeconomic status, emphasizing that healthcare practitioners must understand how these variables can be barriers to the achievement of health.

EDUCATING FUTURE OCCUPATIONAL THERAPY PRACTITIONERS

Considering these multiple factors, what educational experiences can prepare future practitioners to meet these challenges while remaining true to the values and philosophy underlying occupational therapy? How can we educate future practitioners to meet the daunting health-related needs of individuals, organizations, and populations?

Many healthcare-related programs are involved in community-based service-learning projects. It appears that this educational approach, accompanied by calls for service from national and international entities, can begin to solve global problems while simultaneously educating students to be vital community members. You will read narratives and examples of this throughout this book.

In addition to addressing the occupational needs of individuals and society, our educational programs need to increase their focus in other areas as well. The AOTA Centennial Vision and the current and future healthcare environment call for occupational therapy to be a scientifically driven, evidence-based profession. It is the only way to demonstrate that the values and outcomes of our practice make a real difference. Particularly in these times of fiscal scarcity, survival in the healthcare arena depends on evidence to support claims of outcomes we purport to achieve. Calls for documenting the evidence that engaging in occupation promotes wellness and health are a constant din. Such authors as Suarez-Balcazar et al. (2005; 2006), call upon community–university partnerships to be leaders in modeling this research on an ongoing basis. Additionally, an AOTA committee was convened to make recommendations to the profession, focusing on building linkages between research, education, and practice (AOTA, 2007b). Community-based participatory action research is also consistent with the client-centered focus of occupational therapy, whereby the client is viewed as a collaborator.

In order to achieve the goals articulated in the Centennial Vision, one area to consider is education of future leaders in occupational therapy: "The need for leadership in health care has never been greater" (Institute of Medicine, 2001, p. 5). The Kellogg Foundation, in its report "Leadership Reconsidered: Engaging Higher Education in Social Change," identified a *leader* as a person who is prepared to be an agent of positive change in the community. The traditional medical model of training healthcare professionals is no longer adequate to meet the needs of future healthcare providers (Lorenzo et al., 2006). In order to educate students to be leaders, institutions of higher learning must "be engaged in the work of society and the community, modeling effective leadership and problem solving skills, demonstrating how to accomplish change for the common good" (Astin & Astin, 2000, p. 2).

What educational practices can help students acquire these skills? Astin and Astin (2000) report that student involvement in service-learning is one educational strategy that has evidence to support its effectiveness in this area.

In order to educate professionals to fully understand the critical importance of participation and engagement, we must carefully select educational approaches that model these values. Numerous educational pedagogies have been discussed in the occupational therapy literature, including case methods, problem-focused learning, and collaborative learning (Seruya, 2007). Chapter 11 by Patricia Crist in this text offers pedagogical insights as well.

Seifer (1998) reviewed strategies used in medical education programs that included competency training and community-based education. For medical students, community-based education has ushered in positive attitudes toward people from diverse backgrounds. Community-based service-learning improves students' knowledge of community resources and socioeconomic determinants of health. Student knowledge of these factors was even greater when faculty identified community-based education strategies as course outcomes (Seifer, 1998). In South Africa, service to underserved populations is mandatory for all healthcare students. Service-learning helps students understand the power and potential of occupational therapy, while providing a way to work with communities and organizations (Lorenzo et al., 2006).

In many of the chapters in this book you will read how students who engaged in service-learning in their communities developed a greater understanding of *occupation*. This may be the most-compelling argument for community-based coursework.

PROFESSIONAL EDUCATION FOR THE FUTURE

According to Coppard and Dickerson (2007), the term *professional education* describes educational programs that train students to deliver the services of a particular profession. The objectives of these programs should include achievement of competencies defined by the profession, ethical behaviors, and a concern for scholarship. Occupational therapy's professional education goal is to educate a cadre of students who have the skills and competencies to practice in a "changing and dynamic" healthcare delivery system.

Although there are no prescriptive formulas for how to achieve this educational goal, the ACOTE standards do state that the program must be consistent with the mission of the sponsoring institution and with the current philosophy of occupational therapy education. Additionally, the accreditation guidelines for an entry-level master's prepared occupational therapist requires graduates of these programs to acquire basic skills in order to fill the roles of direct care provider, educator, manager, and champion for both the consumer and the profession (ACOTE, 2007). To achieve these educational outcomes, the philosophy of occupational therapy education states that:

> ... educators use active learning that engages the learner in a collaborative process that builds on prior knowledge and experience and integrates professional academic knowledge, experiential learning, clinical reasoning, and self-reflection. Occupational therapy education promotes integration of philosophical and theoretical knowledge, values, beliefs, ethics, and technical skills for broad application to practice in order to improve human participation and quality of life for those individuals with and without impairments and limitations. (AOTA, 2007a, p. 129)

Collectively, the authors and researchers who have contributed to this book have come to the realization that service-learning is a viable and valuable teaching pedagogy that meets the call to service. The global echo from this call reminds us, as occupational therapy educators, of the need to develop change agents for a healthcare environment that must move beyond the medical model and toward partnership to equitably serve those in need.

SERVICE-LEARNING

Service-learning has been defined in many ways, and a quick review of Chapter 1 reacquaints us with the definition we embrace in this text. Philosophically, service-learning is based on education obtained through experiential learning. According to Dewey (1916), education is an active process that involves constant reorganization and reconstruction of past experiences in order to make meaning of present experiences. Similar to the philosophy that underlies occupational therapy educational practice, service-learning promotes learning by doing. This enables students to actively apply classroom theory to community social issues. Learning occurs through an interactive process between students and community partners or clients and action. It is focused on solving community problems while learning academic content. It is a partnership that honors the capacity of human beings to learn by active participation in their environment (Cynkin & Robinson, 1990). Service-learning literature reports that students engaged in community-based service learning overcome their stereotypical thinking about those who are different then they are (Hanc, 2008), increase their ethical awareness (Greene, 1997), and increase their ability to work as members of interdisciplinary teams (Lukasiwicz, 2008).

For example, in Service Learning I, a service-learning class taught at my school, Husson University, students reported in their reflective journals that they felt that service-learning made them more competent to be change agents in their communities. The following student journal entries from Service Learning I examine the interconnectedness of client needs and community limits related to buildings and architecture:

> I am sure that it is frustrating to try to call attention to building problems because they (people with disabilities) may feel they are only calling attention to their disabilities. It seems unfair that as an OT we are trying to help people become more independent, yet they (people with disabilities) cannot socially participate because facilities are not following ADA regulations. By doing these reviews I have seen how important it is to keep the community informed and really make changes to aid our future clients.

> I find that this not only important for occupational therapy students but is information that everyone should be informed with what it takes to make a building accessible. If everyone puts forth the effort in their community then one-by-one we can make a difference and help people in need of their independence!

Reflective journals provide clarity and reinforcement for the experiences and beliefs that students acquire and allow these experiences to be gathered into a coherent whole. Perhaps this is one reason it is a great tool for training occupational therapists. Service-learning literature also reports that that service-learning is most successful if it clearly relates to a students' learning, which is especially important with younger students (Hoppes, Bender, & DeGrace, 2005; Waskiewicz, 2002). In other words, if learning outcomes clearly delineate the reason for participating in the service project, students report being more positive about their service than if they provide service that has no clear learning-related outcomes (Moely, Furco, & Reed, 2008; Hoppes, Bender, & DeGrace, 2005). Moreover, students who participate in community-service projects in schools that clearly articulate a mission of service are more positive about their service experiences. This is nothing new for occupational therapy, because we recognize the importance of context to meaningful and purposeful occupation (AOTA, 2008b).

Although there have been calls for a return to occupational therapy's roots and bedrock values, we still hear grumblings from students entering practice settings and being inculcated into the medical model. Concerns emerge when occupation-based practice is not applied. It can be a threat to communities, our profession, evidence-gathering, and the value of occupation in health promotion. It is interesting to note that innovation theorist Estrin (2009) reports in her book that U.S. schools typically lag behind adopting best educational practices by 25 years. This suggests that we should be ready as educators to enhance our curricula with teaching strategies that will help us transform our practice to what it could and should be. We believe that service-learning is one way that occupational therapists can move toward the vision we have articulated for ourselves in our Frameworks.

Table 2-1 summarizes the fit among service-learning as pedagogy, occupational therapy philosophy, and the ACOTE standards. Table 2-1 will help you see the compatibility among service-learning pedagogy, occupational therapy philosophy, and the ACOTE standards. If applicable, we hope this helps you to design service-learning educational opportunities for your students that integrate these three categories.

Table 2-1 Compatibility Between Service-Learning Pedagogy, OT Philosophy, and the ACOTE Standards.

Service-Learning as Pedagogy	Occupational Therapy Philosophy	ACOTE Standard
Active experiential learning (Learn and Serve America, n.d.)	Engage in meaningful occupation	**B.2.3.** Articulate to consumers, potential employers, colleagues, third-party payers, regulatory boards, policymakers, other audiences, and the general public both the unique nature of occupation as viewed by the profession of occupational therapy and the value of occupation to support participation in context(s) for the client.
"Service-learning combines service objectives with learning objectives . . ." (Learn and Serve America, n.d.). The literature identifies this as a critical element of service-learning so its purpose is relevant to students.	"*Occupation* has been defined as 'Goal-directed pursuits that typically extend over time, have meaning to the performance, and involve multiple tasks'" (AOTA, 2008b, p. 628).	**B.3.5.** Apply theoretical constructs to evaluation and intervention with various types of clients and practice contexts to analyze and effect meaningful occupation.
Service-learning outcomes are more positive when delivered in an environment whose mission supports it (Moely, Furco, & Reed, 2008).	"The term *context* refers to a variety of interrelated conditions that are within and surrounding the client. These interrelated contexts often are less tangible than physical and social environments but nonetheless exert a strong influence on performance" (AOTA, 2008b, p. 642).	**B.2.2.** Explain the meaning and dynamics of occupation and activity, including the interaction of areas of occupation, performance skills, performance patterns, activity demands, context(s), and client factors.

(continued)

Table 2-1 (*Continued*)

Service-Learning as Pedagogy	Occupational Therapy Philosophy	ACOTE Standard
Students and community partners work together to solve community-based problems (Learn and Serve America, n.d.).	"Occupational justice to describe the profession's concern with ethical, moral, and civic factors that can support or hinder health-promoting engagement in occupations and participation in home and community life" (AOTA, 2008a, p. 230).	**B.2.9.** Express support for the quality of life, well-being, and occupation of the individual, group, or population to promote physical and mental health and prevention of injury and disease considering the context (e.g., cultural, physical, social, personal, spiritual, temporal, virtual).
Students collaborate with community partners, recognizing the importance of the community in the learning process (Learn and Serve America, n.d.).	Occupational therapy practitioners develop a collaborative relationship with clients in order to understand their experiences and desires for intervention, . . . The collaborative approach, which is used throughout the process, honors the contributions of the client and the occupational therapy practitioner" (AOTA, 2008b, p. 647).	**B.5.1.** Use evaluation findings based on appropriate theoretical approaches, models of practice, and frames of reference to develop occupation-based intervention plans and strategies (including goals and methods to achieve them) based on the stated needs of the client as well as data gathered during the evaluation process in collaboration with the client and others.
Service-learning involves reflection on service (Learn and Serve America, n.d.).	"Throughout the process, the occupational therapy practitioner is engaged continually in clinical reasoning about the client's engagement in occupation" (AOTA, 2008b, p. 647).	**B.1.2.** Employ logical thinking, critical analysis, problem solving, and creativity.

(*continued*)

Table 2-1 (*Continued*)

Service-Learning as Pedagogy	Occupational Therapy Philosophy	ACOTE Standard
Analyzes and meets complex needs of a community (Learn and Serve America, n.d.).	OT is holistic	**B.2.9.** Express support for the quality of life, well-being, and occupation of the individual, group, or population to promote physical and mental health and prevention of injury and disease considering the context (e.g., cultural, physical, social, personal, spiritual, temporal, virtual).

CONCLUSION

Service-learning's fit with occupational therapy and the occupational therapy educational philosophy can aid us in educating occupational therapy students for the future. In order to accomplish our Centennial Vision, the occupational therapy profession needs to build and evolve its curricula, continue to embrace service-learning, and gather and publish the resultant data to assess these efforts and to look forward. Finally, we must honor the social contract of occupational therapy, which is to ensure that all people, organizations, and populations are able to participate in meaningful occupations of their choosing (Fazio, 2008).

One of the more heartening and serendipitous elements of this work is recognizing how the goals of service-learning seem to parallel the founding thoughts and beliefs of occupational therapy, thus providing a viable educational strategy to achieve our Centennial Vision. The chapters that follow will provide you with examples of how this educational strategy has been successfully integrated into a number of occupational therapy and occupational therapy assistant curricula. We hope you will be as excited as we are by what you read.

References

Accreditation Council for Occupational Therapy Education (ACOTE). (2007). Accreditation standards for a master's-degree-level educational program for the occupational therapist. *American Journal of Occupational Therapy, 61*, 652–661.

American Occupational Therapy Association (AOTA). (2008a). Occupational therapy services in the promotion of health and the prevention of disease and disability. *American Journal of Occupational Therapy, 62*, 694–703.

American Occupational Therapy Association. (2008b). Occupational Therapy Practice, Framework: Domain & Process, 2nd Edition. *American Journal of Occupational Therapy, 62*, 625–683.

American Occupational Therapy Association. (2007a). Philosophy of occupational therapy education. *American Journal of Occupational Therapy, 61*, November–December.

American Occupational Therapy Association. (2007b). Create Better Linkages Between Education, Research and Practice Ad Hoc Committee: Final Report to the Board of Directors. Retrieved online August 23, 2009 from: http://www.aota.org/News/Centennial/AdHoc/2007/40991.aspx.

American Occupational Therapy Association. (2005). Occupational therapy code of ethics (2005). *American Journal of Occupational Therapy, 59*, 639–642.

American Occupational Therapy Association. (2004). Occupational therapy's commitment to nondiscrimination and inclusion. *American Journal of Occupational Therapy, 58*, 668.

Astin, A. W. & Astin, H. S. (2000). Leadership reconsidered: engaging higher education in social change. Retrieved online August 23, 2009 from: http://www.wkkf.org/DesktopModules/WKF.00_DmaSupport/ViewDoc.aspx?fld=PDFFile&CID=148&ListID=28&ItemID=1483368&LanguageID=0

Clark, F. (2006). Moving forward: We have the vision, now let's make it happen. Retrieved September 29, 2008, from http://www.aota.org/News/Centennial/Background/36569.aspx.

Clinton, B. (2007). *Giving: How each of us can change the world.* New York: Knopf.

Community-Campus Partnerships on Health. (2008). Discipline-specific resources, including syllabi. Retrieved November 11, 2008, from http://depts.washington.edu/ccph/servicelearningres.html.

Coppard, B., & Dickerson, A. (2007). A descriptive review of occupational therapy education. *American Journal of Occupational Therapy, 61*, 672–677.

Cynkin, S., & Robinson, A. M. (1990). *Occupational Therapy and Activities Health: Towards Health Through Activities.* Boston: Little, Brown & Co.

Dewey, J. (1916). *Democracy and education: An Introduction to the Philosophy of Education.* New York: The Free Press.

Estrin, J. (2009). *Closing the innovation gap: Reigniting the spark of creativity in a global economy*. New York: McGraw-Hill.

Fazio, L. (2008). *Developing occupation-centered programs for the community* (2nd edition). Upper Saddle River, NJ: Prentice Hall.

Grady, A. P. (1995). Building inclusive community: A challenge for occupational therapy, 1994 Eleanor Clarke Slagle Lecture, *American Journal of Occupational Therapy, 49,* 300–310.

Greene, D. (1997). The use of service learning in client environments to enhance ethical reasoning in students. *American Journal of Occupational Therapy, 51,* 844–852.

Hanc, J. (2008, November 11). Finding similarities among differences. *New York Times,* p. F4.

Hoppes, S., Bender, D., & DeGrace, B. W. (2005). Service learning is a perfect fit for occupational and physical therapy education. *Journal of Allied Health, 34,* 47–50.

Institute of Medicine. (2001). *Crossing the quality chasm: A new health system for the 21st century*. Washington DC: National Academies Press.

Learn and Serve America. (n.d.) What is service learning? Retrieved November 17, 2008, from http://www.servicelearning.org/what_is_service-learning/service-learning_is/index.php.

Lorenzo, T., Duncan, M., Buchanan, H., & Alsop, A. (Eds.). (2006). *Practice and service learning in occupational therapy: enhancing potential in context*. New York: John Wiley & Sons.

Lukasiwicz, M. (2008). Peering into a future of collaboration: A student's insight into interdisciplinary service learning. *OT Practice, 13,* 13–16.

Moely, B., Furco, A., & Reed, J. (2008). Charity and social change: The impact of individual preferences on service learning outcomes. *Michigan Journal of Community Service Learning, 15,* 37–48.

Obama, B. (2007, December 5). Obama issues call to serve, vows to make national service important cause of his presidency. Mt. Vernon, Iowa. Retrieved online November 10, 2008, from http://www.barackobama.com/2007/12/05/obama_issues_call_to_serve_vow.php.

Reilly, M. (1962). Occupational therapy can be one of the great ideas of twentieth-century medicine. *American Journal of Occupational Therapy, 16,* 2–9.

Scharmer, C. O. (2007). *Theory U: Leading from the future as it emerges. The social technology of presencing*. Retrieved November 17, 2008, from http://www.theoryu.com/documents/TU-ch00intro.pdf.

Seifer, S. D. (1998). Recent and emerging trends in undergraduate medical education—curricular responses to a rapidly changing health care system. *West Journal of Medicine, 168,* 400–411.

Seruya, F. (2007). Preparing entry-level occupational therapy students: An examination of current teaching practices. *Education Special Interest Section Quarterly, 17*, 1-4.

Suarez-Balcazar, Y., Munoz, J., & Fisher, G. (2006). Building culturally competent community–university partnerships for occupational therapy scholarship. In Gary Keihofner (Ed.), *Research in occupational therapy: Methods of inquiry for enhancing practice.* Philadelphia: F. A. Davis.

Suarez-Balcazar, Y., Hammel, J., Helfrich, C., Thomas, J., Wilson, T., & Head-Ball, D. (2005). A model of university–community partnerships for occupational therapy scholarship and practice. *Occupational Therapy in Health Care, 19,* 47-70.

Waskiewicz, R. (2002). Impact of service learning on occupational therapy students' awareness of, commitment to, and sense of responsibility toward community. Master of Arts thesis, Temple University, Philadelphia, Pennsylvania. 197 pages; AAT 3040370.

Wilcock, A. (2006). *An Occupational Perspective of Health.* Thorofare, NJ: Slack.

World Health Report. (2007). A safer future: global public health security in the twenty-first century. Retrieved October 2, 2008, from http://www.who.int/whr/2007/overview/en/index.html.

Chapter 3

Who Sits at the Head of the Table? A Reflection on Community, Student, and Faculty Partnerships

Beth P. Velde, PhD, OTR/L, Doris T. Davis, and Gary R. Grant

Here it is, the first day of our service-learning partnership. We walk into the Tillery Community Center, two faculty and four students. Community members are milling around. A long, rectangular table with chairs is in the center of the room—the obvious space for our meeting. As faculty, we quickly realize that if we are to create a partnership with this community, we must begin now. Where should the six of us sit? If we all sit together, will it seem like "us and them"? If one of us sits at the head of the table, would this be perceived as a position of power and control? The students are likely to sit in a row right next to each other. How will this be viewed by community members—will the students be seen as weak, uncomfortable, or fearful?

As faculty, we decide to meet quickly with our students to talk, to provide the students with some guidance regarding our expectations, and to remind them that, like the community residents, they know each other but not members of the "other" group. We talk about how they felt the first day of class and ask them what helped make them feel welcome. The students decide they need to split up and introduce themselves to community residents and ask the residents to give them a tour of the center. This feels more like what we intended.

Next, we tackle the table issue. Quickly we meet with our community partners and ask if we can use the round table. Of course, they say— we just wanted to make sure everyone had enough room. We now alert the students that they need to "split up" and intersperse among the community residents, faculty, and students.

Later, we talk as a large group—students, faculty, and community— about how this beginning influenced the way we perceived each other. Our discussion focuses on collaboration and partnerships. We realize that no one partner sits at the head of the table; we each share responsibility for leading the project. Because we approached this first meeting with mindfulness, we set the stage for building a partnership.

The authors of this chapter represent the community organizations and faculty involved in our partnership. In this chapter, we have consciously chosen to speak in the personal—to use, we, as a representation of our partnership. We have learned to trust and respect each other. This chapter is our story, what has worked for us.

Researchers have identified five fundamental elements for effective service-learning: placement quality, application between classroom and community, reflection, diversity, and listening to the community's voice (Honnet & Poulsen, 1989). In considering these five elements, we believe that the role of the partners within each component is essential to the success of service-learning. A clear understanding of the roles and activities can enhance the service-learning experiences for everyone involved. We are involved in an 11-year service-learning endeavor involving a university occupational therapy (OT) department, two "grassroots" community organizations, and residents of a crossroads community in rural eastern North Carolina. The purpose of our chapter is to explain what has made our experience successful and to analyze available literature (especially occupational therapy) for evidence from other successful partnerships.

Educational experiences that include an experiential component with active application of course or curricular knowledge to real-life community problems are considered service-learning (Eyler & Giles, 1999). According to Seifer (1998), all partners in the experience prepare for and reflect on both the service and the learning, and the nature of the experience is reciprocal in terms of relationships and benefits. But what roles do the partners play, and what activities contribute to reciprocity?

ROLES OF THE CAMPUS PARTNERS

Establishing partnerships with communities can occur in several ways. At the organizational level, universities and colleges, as part of their mission, philosophy, and strategic plan, support and encourage service-learning. Institution-wide professional development prepares faculty for their roles and the skills to carry out needed activities. The university or college may have a service-learning center that seeks community organizations, conducts community needs assessments, establishes agreements, negotiates for placements, and sets global (not course-specific) goals and outcomes. The center brings together interested parties for education, networking, and celebrations. Departments and instructors interested in incorporating service-learning work with the center. The center may assist instructors in integrating service-learning into syllabi, developing course-specific goals and outcome assessments, determining credit for the experience, and mentoring faculty in the scholarship of engagement. Center staff may provide mentors or coaches for faculty new to service-learning. In the initial stages of our project, the university was in the discussion stage regarding the development of a university service-learning center, and we did not have the resources provided by university centers.

An instructor can also initiate service-learning. The instructor reviews the mission and philosophy of the institution and department to ensure that service-learning is congruent with the institution. This congruence provides a basis for the instructor to request resources needed for service-learning, such as instructor time for negotiation with communities, course-planning time, student orientation, transportation, and so on. The instructor establishes clear goals and objectives that link the course content to community service. The goals and objectives assist the instructor in identifying appropriate community service opportunities, taking into account the strengths and needs of the students and the community.

When deciding to identify a community partnership without the support of a centralized center, the instructor needs to consider the following:

1. Is there congruence between the community's vision, the instructor's vision, and the course goals related to service-learning?
2. Is there a willingness to collaborate regarding the student/faculty roles and community services provided?
3. Can trust and respect be established between the partners?
4. Are there reciprocal benefits for all partners? (Gitlow & Flecky, 2005)
5. Is there potential for establishing effective methods of communication?
6. Can the partners build a plan for entering and exiting the community?

As the faculty member who was the campus partner, I reflected on my role and my beliefs about working with the community. How could I establish trust and mutual respect? What did *reciprocity* mean when the partners were faculty, students, and the community, with the two latter groups in a traditionally less powerful position? How could I equalize power among the partners so that we recognized each other's strengths and needs? I decided that during each encounter with one of the groups, I would approach the encounter with questions, not demands. For example, when approaching the community health advisory committee, I asked about the health concerns they felt were most pressing in the community and why they felt these health issues existed. When approaching a student group for the first time, I asked them to describe "community" and to reflect on communities they belonged to. I reflected on my own skills and asked my partners to do the same. During our monthly meetings, we shared these skills with each other. In time, we felt comfortable sharing our weaknesses and supporting each other in developing our weaknesses into strengths.

For example, at first I was hesitant to share my lack of knowledge of Black history. I worried about how I would be viewed by my African American partners. Would they think I didn't care, would they think I was ignorant? During meetings in the community, I quickly learned that one of the partners taught using stories. I became increasingly comfortable asking questions during his stories. I began to understand the history of naming individuals and its relationship to slavery, the power of land ownership, and the environmental injustices People of Color experience. My questions led to discussions about the role of occupational therapy in dealing with social and environmental injustices. From these discussions, we determined a plan for a student orientation that would include community educators who could help students place the community and its residents in a historical context.

I thought about activities that would provide reflective experiences for both my students and my community partners to address power issues. For example, students were asked to think about and record the terms used to refer to occupational therapy participants in traditional clinical settings. They were asked to remember times when they observed health interactions in these traditional settings. We wrote these terms on the white board and talked about each—not in a value-laden manner, but analytically. For example, we did not label some as "good" ways to refer to occupational therapy participants and some as "bad." Instead, we tried to describe the terms as a way to describe roles and relationships. They came up with "patient," "client," "hip patient in 232," "the schizophrenic," "Beth," and so on. As the group facilitator, I guided the discussion to evaluate: the impact of the health system; cultural norms; historical uses of racist, classicist, and gendered language; and ageist perspectives. The goal was to try and understand how we choose words and phrases to refer to the persons we work with. We contrasted each term with an alternative. For example, we looked at the contrast between "patient" and "agent" and "consumer" and "client." When we went to the community, residents talked about names and the history of naming slaves. They talked about the difference between being addressed by Mr. or Mrs., by their first name, or by "Miss Beth." This conversation illustrated the role of power in the process of naming; for example, the power of the slave owner over a slave's name. The community residents helped students understand they needed to start with a formal name (e.g., "Mrs. Velde") and wait until the resident informed the student if he or she could use "Miss Beth" or "Beth." Students also thought about and discussed what they would like to be called as an occupational therapist. This led to a discussion of name tags, what should go on their nametags, when to wear nametags, the symbolic meaning of nametags, and the value of having occupational therapy and participant nametags that are the same (materials, quality, size, etc.) as a visual way to equalize power relationships.

ROLES OF COMMUNITY PARTNERS

Increasingly, communities are becoming cognizant of the power issues surrounding community–campus partnerships. They actively seek campus partnerships to address their health needs through service-learning because of the reciprocal nature of such experiences. Our partnership was initiated at the community's request. The motto of our university is "To serve," and we are known for our service to the community. The community had the following Statement of Philosophy and Vision of Health:

> The Concerned Citizens of Tillery (CCT) and the CCT Area Wide Health Committee hold that access to good health care is a basic human right, and the denial of this right is unjust. We hold that the promotion of good health requires **educational, social, economic, political, spiritual, occupational, and environmental approaches** in addition to traditional health care service. We further hold that the confrontation of racism, sexism, and all other "isms" at every level is a basic step toward a holistic health care which heals as well as prevents illnesses.
>
> Besides providing for the immediate needs of the community, another of our purposes is to develop a just and effective health movement. It is the first responsibility of a just health system to take directions from the community and the priorities it establishes.

CCT is committed to **assuring that those who work in collaboration and/or partnership with CCT learn** about the conditions that contribute to poor health, and develop the skills and the sensitivity needed to address these conditions. CCT hopes that those who participate with us, along with our youth, will learn about career options, which will enable them to address these problems in the future.

This philosophy and vision provided the basis for collaboration and negotiation between the university faculty members, the community, and the community organizations. According to Williams, "partnerships consist of organizations that have their own mission, goals and work plans. A successful service-learning partnership is collaborative in nature compelled to come together by a shared vision. The collaborative must create a shared mission and function using creativity, compromise, and thinking outside the box—leaving their organizational egos behind" (Reep, L'Esperance, Williams, Jones, & Voelp, 2008). In light of that, our mission was as follows:

The conditions needed for good health include recreational facilities, excellent schools and medical facilities, lifelong learning opportunities, nutritious food, and economic development. These will not be granted by outside institutions, but will be created by a strong community working in equal partnership with other groups. This partnership believes that an understanding of discrimination, institutional racism and the cultural values of communities engaged in the struggle for human rights and self-determination helps students and faculty understand their own society and prepares them to work in diverse communities in partnership with social change organizations. We will actively engage in activities that develop such understanding. Ending environmental degradation of the poor and people of color decreases Black land loss and promotes economic development and self-sufficiency. Together, ECU and CCT help citizens participate in cultural, educational and political activities that are a central part of CCT's agenda to achieve community health through social change. ECU students facilitate engagement by empowering citizens to create and adapt physical, political, temporal, and sociocultural environments.

Our service-learning project has a dual focus on community needs and student/faculty learning; our relationship is reciprocal in nature and built on trust and respect. Our partnership has withstood the test of changing membership, grants that have come and gone, an occupational therapy educational program that has transitioned to a Masters of Science program, and changing priorities at the university. The occupational therapy faculty use a community-built practice model. According to Wittman and Velde (2001b), community-built practice is interactive and collaborative with occupational therapy participants, works with both the community's strengths and needs, focuses on prevention and wellness using a holistic perspective of health, and ends when the community has built the capacity for empowerment. It is framed in a perspective of social justice that addresses both occupational and environmental justice. Hansen et al. (2007) claim that service-learning framed in a justice perspective can help "students learn how social responsibility calls them to address these conditions through encounter and action" (p. 33).

From the beginning, the two community organizations served as the drivers of the service-learning process. This has continued throughout our relationship. During monthly meetings, representatives from the community, community organizations, and the university faculty discuss community issues that are jointly identified. The agendas for these meetings are developed first by the community and then shared with other partners for additional agenda items. From the issues, the group develops goals that address both community needs and student/faculty learning. The occupational therapy faculty present a menu of occupational therapy skills, programs, and research they can offer. The community asks questions and presents issues and concerns about the options, and together the partners choose the experiences. Types of service-learning experiences have included research about health and quality of life, home health services, group programs, community education sessions, and consultation with health clinic staff.

Communication is a key to trust and respect. As partners, we use e-mail, phone calls, face-to-face meetings, and occasionally letters to share information. When we use e-mail, we copy all partners on the correspondence. Sebastian et al. (2002) also found that e-mail was an efficient method of maintaining information flow. Minutes of face-to-face meetings are distributed to all partners. Grant reports are mutually developed and edited. Whenever possible, manuscripts and conference presentations are mutually developed, and, when it is appropriate, there is joint authorship. Face time provides opportunities for showing concern for all partners. Face time requires physically being in the community—for meetings, for students' time in the community. As faculty, we learned that we needed to stay for the entire partners' meeting, not just the portion that dealt with occupational therapy. Whenever possible, students attend partners' meetings. We also learned that attending important community events, such as celebrations, club meetings, and funerals, helps to build trust and respect.

EXAMPLES OF PARTNERSHIP ACTIVITIES

Goals and associated outcomes have varied. For example, in 1997 the community presented concerns about the lack of knowledge regarding the health of its residents. Occupational therapy, health education, nursing and medical faculty, and students used the SF-36, with additional questions focused on occupations, to conduct a door-to-door health survey of the community, supported by a Learn and Serve America grant (Shah & Glascoff, 1998). From the survey results, the partners identified the need for health education and home health services. When the Learn and Serve grant ended, the occupational therapy service-learning experience continued with resources from both the university and the community. According to our community partners, "Sticking around to address community issues" is an important component in building trust.

In 2004, occupational therapy and epidemiology students and faculty from East Carolina University and the University of North Carolina at Chapel Hill repeated the door-to-door survey. We included additional questions about the environment because of community concerns regarding commercial hog operations, pulp mill operations, heating and air conditioning systems used by community residents, and the presence of mold and mildew. From these survey results, the partners identified the need to focus on issues of environmental injustice and the negative impact it has on human health. Occupational therapy students and faculty provided community and home safety assessments, falls prevention education, and wellness programs with the support of a grant from the National Institute of Environmental Health Sciences (NIEHS) that was co-authored by the partners. The partners hold monthly meetings about the grant and discuss the occupational therapy services, environmental justice projects, and research projects related to health. During these discussions they identify issues and needs that could be addressed using service-learning experiences. The university faculty learned to flex with the community's agenda.

The meetings rotate locations, with each partner hosting at least two meetings a year. This is an important symbolic representation of equality among members. Minutes are recorded and circulated, allowing members of the partnership not in attendance to understand the discussion. Discussions at these meetings are open and honest and enhance the quality of the service-learning placements and provide opportunities for reflections by both community and faculty.

We believe that campus–community partnerships are strengthened when the university doesn't come to "save" the population, but rather to participate equally in learning and service. We share the principles for effective partnerships published by the Alaska OCS and Tribal Safety Assessment Project (n.d.):

> **Mutual Respect**
> Equality of participation.
> At least one tribal partner must be involved in all discussions.
> Workgroup leads must share all relevant information with all members.
>
> **Open and Honest Communication**
> Feel free to express disagreement.
> Express disagreement in a respectful manner.
>
> **Consistent Participation: A commitment to continue through the process, willingness to think in new ways, recognition and acknowledgements of commonalities**

Consensus in decisions.
Shared decision-making.
Flexibility.

Accommodation of Individual Differences

Remember, we work across cultures.
Be sensitive to different thinking processes (when asking a question, count to 10 before deciding that no one is going to respond).
Be aware of differences in what constitutes politeness and social norms.
Remember, not everyone understands the acronyms, don't assume.

Beck and Barnes (2007) also discuss the potential imbalance of power between institutions of higher education and other agencies. Within their service-learning experience, they addressed power issues and developed methods to increase ownership for all involved. We believe that intensive community involvement in both the planning and implementation of student preparation and education phases increases ownership. However, students must also be invested and issues of power between faculty and students and the community and students must be addressed honestly if students are to "buy in."

ROLES OF STUDENT PARTNERS

Service-learning encourages active participation by student partners. This contributes to a feeling of belonging and responsibility. Students in our partnership are required to prepare for each service-learning encounter by accessing resources, determining personal goals for learning, and meeting with involved faculty. They attend orientations on campus and in the community. Campus orientations are intended to increase their understanding of the community's history and culture and to create opportunities for students and faculty to identify biases and assumptions. The majority of our occupational therapy students are young Caucasian females. Our community site is composed of African American elders. Both the faculty and the community organizations carefully plan this cross-cultural encounter.

It allows our students to move away from a "wall of academic isolation" (Hoppes, Bender, & DeGrace, 2005, p. 49) and into a community setting with diversity in terms of race, socioeconomic status, and culture.

One piece of our orientation is the discussion of "community." We use active learning strategies to analyze the concept. For example, students are asked to use supplies and materials to construct a community. Typically, these constructions include schools, churches, houses, roads, grocery stores, entertainment centers, hospitals, shops, and restaurants. They discuss their creations together with faculty. They identify sources for their knowledge of community and describe their own experiences with community. With directed questioning, they discuss roles of community members and occupations in rural communities. They talk about their knowledge of African American communities and of African American history. They then visit our service-learning site, where our community partners begin their educational role. At the site, community residents share the history of their community, discuss slavery and sharecropping, show examples of Resettlement homes and programs, and talk about the practice of naming during slavery. Students go on a tour of the community conducted by a community member. Finally, they compare their on-campus experience with their community experience. Community members and faculty are present to support the students and to honestly reflect on aspects of culture and history that impact both occupations and health. Follow-up sessions use guided, reciprocal peer-questioning techniques to have students critically reflect about health in rural areas and their roles as occupational therapists. For example, questions might include, "What are the differences between health services in urban areas and the rural area you visited?", "How are the older adults you spoke with similar to or different from your grandparents?", "What are the strengths and weaknesses of providing occupational therapy services in a community versus in a clinic?", and "How is community occupational therapy assessment related to the individual occupational therapy assessment process that we studied during intervention courses?"

Students are expected to listen to community members and to collaboratively plan goals for occupational therapy interventions.

Community members are considered experts in terms of their lifestyle, and students/faculty are experts in terms of occupational therapy practice. For example, during a presentation on falls and fear of falling, students presented fall education posters obtained from a national government agency. Community members were quick to reject the efficacy of the posters for this community, pointing out that the photographs featured Caucasian elders, not African American elders. The context of the photographs was not congruent with the predominant context of community residents who reside in rural areas in mobile homes or in small single-family dwellings. Students and community members discussed the issue and decided that the students should return the posters to the agency with a letter explaining the cultural and racial issues.

After each interaction, students complete documentation about the interaction and share these with the participants. They talk together about the student perceptions of the interaction and the community member's perception. Students reflect on the service-learning experiences in three ways: verbally through meetings with faculty and community, in photographs and drawings, and through journals. We found that structured reflections work better. The following are two examples of student-reflection prompts:

> Close your eyes and replay your experience in Tillery. Retrace the sequence; recall your significant thoughts, feelings, team and participant interactions, objects, culture, and physical environment. Draw or write about the highlights of this experience. Reflect upon the highlights you recorded and report your observations.

> Haiku is a form of poetry through which you express yourself and your impressions of the world. Begin by naming the intervention experience you had today. Now, describe it. Name the setting, describe the setting. Then describe the feelings you have about the image. Now, go back through what you've written and underline the key words and phrases that really describe the essence of the experience. Move these around and play with them in your mind until there are only seven syllables: one line of five syllables, one of seven syllables, and another line of five syllables. (Wittman & Velde, 2001a, p. 29)

Our students report positive and long-lasting impacts of this service-learning experience (Velde, Wittman, & Mott, 2007) and consider it a quality experience. We do this by ensuring that a faculty member and a community partner are present for each interaction in the community. Students observe the partners model trusting relationships. Student ownership of the service-learning experience is built by providing safe learning experiences with increasing levels of responsibility. One student stated,

> I think I learned to trust myself more 'cause when I first came into the program I had self-esteem issues and was a little bit worried about coming out of my shell and being myself, speaking in general, and being here and being able to relate to new individuals . . . So it was an enlightening experience and it put a lot of love into my heart for this community. (Velde, Wittman, & Mott, 2007, p. 86)

The experience helped students "hear their stories from a different perspective and we have to learn how to understand it from their point of view and learn to really appreciate what is being said" (Velde, Wittman, & Mott, 2007, p. 86). Students felt this understanding was fostered because, "Here it was stepping into someone else's home turf" (p. 86).

Hamel (2001) described the impact of interdisciplinary service-learning experiences (physical and occupational therapy, speech and language therapy, exercise physiology) that addressed the needs of homeless elders. Situated in homeless shelters in the Boston area, the students developed a greater awareness regarding cultural issues, political issues, and service issues after the experience. These students expressed an interest in advocacy as a result of their experience. In addition, Hamel found that students increased rapport-building, communication, and programming skills. Gupta (2006) reported on interdisciplinary service-learning in a homeless shelter in Minnesota. Student journals supported changes in students' attitudes, reflection on personal values, and a desire to advocate for participants' needs. Findings from both of these studies are congruent with our research regarding our service-learning experience.

Lohman and Aitken (2002) indicate that not all service-learning experiences result in positive changes in student perceptions. The level of organization at the service-learning site impacts the students' experience. In the experience described by Lohman and Aitken, students at sites that were the most organized reported higher levels of satisfaction and after the experience remained more positive about service-learning. Students who were at disorganized sites were less satisfied with the experience and changed from high agreement to agreement regarding the impact of service-learning on their education. Sebastian et al. (2002) noted a similar finding, with students' altruistic behavior increasing in year three of their experience and knowledge scores showing no significant increase. They hypothesize that the pre and post assessments may not have been sensitive enough to measure change in knowledge. This raises an important issue for service-learning: Do we have effective tools to measure changes in knowledge and skills in service-learning experiences?

Our students learn to listen to the community and to ask many questions regarding the community's needs. Together with faculty, they provide a "menu" of specific occupational therapy interventions that could match the service needs identified by the faculty and community organizations and then let the program participants decide which services to offer. Past student-led services have included a wellness program for elders (Barnard et al., 2004), interdisciplinary occupational therapy and physical therapy home health services (Wittman, Conner-Kerr, Templeton, & Velde, 1999), and occupational therapy services for older women (Velde et al., 2003). The intervention strategies selected by the program participants included activities in the spiritual, cognitive, and physical domains. Each of these programs included outcome evaluations that addressed both service goals and community needs. The results were shared with the community organizations and used to plan new programs.

IDENTIFYING IMPACT ON STUDENTS, FACULTY, AND COMMUNITY

The impact of service-learning on students is identified in many ways. We ask students to read through the goals of the course associated with the service-learning experience. Each student develops goals. These goals are placed on a white board, and the faculty member facilitates a discussion that results in consensus on the overall student-determined goals. To determine if goals are met, we use focus groups, students' journals, facilitated discussions, surveys, and self-efficacy instruments that are oriented to both occupational therapy skills and cultural competence.

Community partners are asked to identify outcomes from the community perspective, and the community staff solicits verbal feedback from residents and program participants.

Faculty have specific goals related to the course content. For our service-learning, community partners debrief faculty during regular meetings and the course-specific goals are discussed. Faculty outcomes are also measured in terms of scholarship products such as presentations and articles. Recently, such engaged scholarship (Suarez-Balcazar et al., 2005) has been recognized by university tenure and promotion criteria and the Carnegie Classification for Community Engagement that recognizes universities that collaborate with communities "for the mutually beneficial exchange of knowledge and resources in a context of partnership and reciprocity" (Carnegie Foundation, 2007, p. 1).

Gitlow and Flecky (2005) described a multi-method assessment matrix. Borrowing from qualitative methodology, the data for multi-method assessments include a variety of sources (community organizations, community participants, students, faculty) with different types of data. Data types include surveys, journals, focus groups, interviews, self-efficacy assessments completed by students, student portfolios, and so on. The matrix includes the identified outcomes with the assessment data. In our experience, the development of the outcomes must involve all partners. Although we have not used a matrix in our service-learning, we see that entering the student, faculty, and community goals in one column with assessment data in consecutive columns would provide a comprehensive perspective of the effectiveness of the service-learning experience, and we anticipate trying this method in the coming year.

WHEN IS IT TIME TO LEAVE A
SERVICE-LEARNING EXPERIENCE?

As partners, we debate whether a service-learning experience continues forever. While I have been in Tillery, the community has told other university researchers and service providers to leave. The community did this when the university partners began to dictate research and service—to act paternalistic and authoritarian. The community indicated that when faculty put their needs above the community's needs, when faculty fail to acknowledge the equal participation of the community, or when the community is able to meet its own needs—then a service-learning partnership may dissolve.

Partnerships end when the university partner withdraws. We have experienced the loss of service-learning when faculty leave because grant money disappears. If service-learning is dependent on grant funding, then a careful plan must be developed to prepare for the end of programs supported by service learning. Otherwise, we believe it becomes even more difficult for communities to establish trust and respect for university partners.

Sometimes faculty discontinue service-learning when a site does not provide quality educational experiences. This lack of quality may result from community organizations that simply do not have the time to spend developing on-site activities because they are stretched in trying to meet their community's needs. Faculty often exacerbate the situation by sending students alone to service-learning experiences, expecting the community to do all of the supervision. Abravanel (n.d.) indicates that staff in community partnerships often feel that service-learning may add to their already overloaded schedule. We believe that faculty must model the behaviors they want their students to portray, and this can only be done if the faculty are on site for at least part of the service-learning experience. Successful service-learning takes a commitment of time from all partners.

Other university partners in our community have dropped our site because of "pragmatic issues," such as the physical distance between the community and the university. Abravanel (n.d.) notes that schedules are one of these pragmatic issues. Communities want programs offered when their constituents are available—nights or weekends for example. Universities want student engagement during class hours or during the semester/quarter, but not during school breaks. Unfortunately, small, rural communities who are in the most need frequently are 60 miles or more away from the closest university. Student and faculty schedules may inhibit these communities from benefiting from service-learning. As partners, we are 60 miles apart. Grant funding helps with mileage costs, avoiding another barrier discussed by Abravanel (n.d.), and creative student scheduling creates a day without classes so that students and faculty can travel and spend the day. Without administrative support to create this schedule, our students could not have participated in this experience. Finding faculty and administrators who are willing to be creative and flexible is essential for service-learning to work in rural areas. According to one of our community partners, "the community would say not enough faculty have this flexibility for they are concerned with their own daily life."

KEEPING THE DREAM ALIVE

Whereas faculty offer the solid connection between the community and the university, students come and go at the end of the semester or upon graduation. Yet we have learned that for our students, dreams have been accomplished and the goals achieved have had a lasting impact on their personal and professional lives. Faculty and universities too often are in control of the presence or absence of service-learning in the community. For our partnerships, we know it is only the community that "stays." It is the community that ultimately defines the success of the dreams and goals on a broader scope as the campus partners come and go. If the next administrator or faculty member is not inclined to make the effort, then the community's dreams and goals have to be renegotiated, and not always successfully. University partners, who control the resources of faculty and students, must be aware of the enormous responsibility they hold when negotiating service-learning.

Why have we been successful for 11 years? We believe it is because we have addressed the five fundamental elements for effective service learning: placement quality, application between classroom and community, reflection, diversity, and listening to the community's voice (Honnet & Poulsen, 1989). We have enhanced placement quality by making sure there is congruence between the university and community organizations' missions and visions; we have collaboratively constructed partnership mission; we provide on-site faculty and community partner supervision; and we hold regular meetings to maintain communication. Together we make sure there is application between classroom and community by considering the impact of our language and we model our services on community-built practice. All partners engage in reflection, separately and together. We maintain diversity in the roles we each assume; the race, ethnicity, gender, and age of our partners and participants; and the historical context framing each of our lives. Above all we listen to the community's voice and have learned to flex with community and "stick around" despite the challenges.

REFERENCES

Abravanel, S. A. (n.d.). *Building community through service-learning: The role of the community partner*. ECS Issue Paper. Denver, CO: ECS.

Alaska OCS and Tribal Safety Assessment Project (n.d.). Principles for effective partnerships. Retrieved February 1, 2008, from http://209.85.165.104/search?q=cache:IXN9NG66hF0J:https://dbh-sweb.state.ak.us/sites/DBH/ocsSafetyAssessment/Document%2520Library3/1/Guidelines%2520for%2520an%2520Authentic%2520Partnership.doc+%22authentic+partnership%22&hl=en&ct=clnk&cd=6&gl=us&client=safari.

Barnard, S., Dunn, S., Reddic, E., Rhodes, K., Russell, J., Tuitt, T., et al. (2004). Wellness in Tillery: A community-built program. *Family and Community Health, 27*, 151–157.

Beck, A. J., & Barnes, K. J. (2007). Reciprocal service-learning: Texas border Head Start and master of occupational therapy students. *Occupational Therapy in Health Care, 21*(1/2), 7–23.

Carnegie Foundation. (2007). *Elective classification: Community engagement: 2008 Documentation Framework*. Stanford, CA: Author.

Eyler, J., & Giles, D. E. (1999). *Where is the service in service learning?* San Francisco, CA: Jossey-Bass.

Gitlow, L., & Flecky, K. (2005). Integrating disability studies concepts into occupational therapy education using service learning. *American Journal of Occupational Therapy, 59*, 546–553.

Gupta, J. (2006). A model for interdisciplinary service-learning experience for social change. *Journal of Physical Therapy Education, 20,* 55-60.

Hamel, P. C. (2001). Interdisciplinary perspectives, service leaning and advocacy: A nontraditional approach to geriatric rehabilitation. *Topics in Geriatric Rehabilitation, 17,* 53-70.

Hansen, A. M. W., Munoz, J., Crist, P. A., Gupta, J., Ideishi, R. I., Primeau, L. A., et al. (2007). Service learning: Meaningful, community-centered professional skill development for occupational therapy students. *Occupational Therapy in Health Care, 21*(1/2), 25-49.

Honnet, E. P., & Poulsen, S. (1989). *Principles of good practice in combining service and learning. Wingspread special report.* Racine, WI: Johnson Foundation.

Hoppes, S., Bender, D., & DeGrace, B. W. (2005). Service learning is a perfect fit for occupational and physical therapy education. *Journal of Allied Health, 34,* 47-50.

Lohman, H., & Aitken, M. J. (2002). Occupational therapy students' attitudes toward service learning. *Physical & Occupational Therapy in Geriatrics, 20*(3/4), 155-264.

Reep, B., L'Esperance, M., Williams, M., Jones, J., & Voelp, R. (2008, March 25). Summer Significance Academy. Paper presented at the East Carolina University 5th Annual Service Learning Conference.

Sebastian, J. G, Skelton, J., Hall, L. A., Assell, R. A., McCollum, B. D., West, K. P., et al. (2002). Interdisciplinary service-learning: A model for community partnership University of Kentucky. In S. D. Seifer , K. Connors, and T. Seifer (Eds.), *Service-learning in health profession education: Case studies from the health professions schools in Service to the Nation Program.* San Francisco: Community-Campus Partnerships for Health. Retrieved April 15, 2008, from http://depts.washington.edu/ccph/pdf_files/Case-kentucky.pdf.

Seifer, S. D. (1998). Service learning: Community campus partnerships for health professions education. *Academic Medicine, 73,* 273-277.

Shah, N., & Glascoff, M. (1998). The Community as classroom: Service-learning in Tillery, North Carolina. In J. S. Noreck, C. Connolly, J. Loerner, & E. Zlotkowhski (Eds.), *Caring and community: Concepts and models for service learning in nursing* (pp. 111-117). Washington, DC: American Association for Higher Education.

Suarez-Balcazar, Y., Hammel, J., Helfrich, C., Thomas, J., Wilson, T., & Head-Ball, D. (2005). A model of university–community partnerships for occupational therapy scholarship. *Occupational Therapy in Health Care, 21*(1/2), 47-70.

Velde, B. P., Wittman, P. P., & Mott, V. (2007). Hands-on learning in Tillery. *Journal of Transformative Education, 5*(1), 79-92.

Velde, B. P., Wittman, P. P., Lee, H., Lee, C., Broadhurst, E., & Caines, M. (2003). Quality of life of older African American women in rural North Carolina. *Journal of Women and Aging, 15*(4), 69-82.

Wittman, P. P., & Velde, B. P. (2001a). Helping occupational therapy students and faculty develop cultural competence. *Occupational Therapy in Health Care, 13*(3/4), 23–32.

Wittman, P. P., & Velde, B. P. (2001b). Occupational therapy in the community: What, why and how. *Occupational Therapy in Health Care, 13*(3/4), 1–5.

Wittman, P., Conner-Kerr, T., Templeton, M. S., & Velde, B. (1999). The Tillery Project: An experience in an interdisciplinary, rural health care service setting. *Physical & Occupational Therapy in Geriatrics, 17*(1), 17–28.

Chapter 4

Cross-Cultural Service-Learning: An Introduction and Best Practices

Joy D. Doll, OTD, OTR/L

Culture is dynamic, is difficult to define, and is everywhere. As the United States becomes more diverse, the impact of culture will continue to complicate human interactions, and healthcare practitioners will be expected to perform in a culturally diverse world (Beach et al., 2005; Black & Wells, 2007). The literature tells us that a lack of cultural awareness leads to breakdowns in communication, poor practitioner–patient rapport, and medical errors (Black & Wells, 2007; Chiang & Carlson, 2003; Spector, 2004). Healthcare providers are expected to attain cultural competence and be capable of interacting with a diverse population (Tseng & Streltzer, 2008). However, preparing students for a diverse world is challenging, and teaching culture in a classroom removes many of the dynamics that impact cross-cultural encounters.

Culture is complicated. Multiple definitions and theoretical approaches towards providing culturally appropriate care exist across the healthcare literature (Rudman & Dennhardt, 2008). Obviously, the variations in definitions of *culture* and approaches to exploring culturally relevant practice make teaching culture a significant challenge. Service-learning provides a model for introducing the concepts of culture in a real-world situation, forcing students to face their personal challenges and to develop the skills necessary to interact in a diverse world. In this chapter, the author will present service-learning as pedagogy for teaching the skills needed in cross-cultural settings. Prior to exploring the role of service-learning in teaching cross-cultural skills important terminology and cultural competence models will be discussed.

WHAT IS CULTURE?

Culture can be defined as "the customary beliefs, social forms, and material traits of a racial, religious, or social group; the set of shared attitudes, values, goals, and practices that characterizes a company or corporation" (Mish, 2008). Culture provides a basis for human beings to create and share meaning (Helman, 2001). The meanings associated with culture drive what humans choose to do and determine life choices. Culture defines the roles and responsibilities of human beings, helping people to know how to respond to life situations. Culture is learned based on experience within the context of the culture permeating both the individual and the environment (Spector, 2004).

In occupational therapy, culture influences occupational engagement, impacting not only which occupations humans choose to engage in but also how they engage in these occupations. Participation in occupations is directly affected by one's culture (Bonder, Martin, & Miracle, 2002). Engagement in occupation is also necessary for health. If occupations are culturally driven, then occupational therapy practitioners have a role in understanding the dynamic interplay between culture and occupation (Wilcock, 2006; Black & Wells, 2007).

In the Occupational Therapy Practice Framework (OTPF), *culture* is defined as

> ...customs, beliefs, activity patterns, behavior standards, and expectations accepted by the society of which the client is a member. Includes ethnicity and values as well as political

aspects, such as laws that affect access to resources and affirm personal rights. Also includes opportunities for education, employment, and economic support. (AOTA, 2008, p. 645)

According to the OTPF, culture is a component of the client's context that "refers to a variety of interrelated conditions that are within and surrounding the client" (AOTA, 2008, p. 645). Culture not only influences the individual, but also the formation of cultural groups. The OTPF refers to cultural groups as being as small as families and as large as ethnic groups. Similarly, Black and Wells (2007) identify that culture influences occupational choices of the person, the professional, society, and the globe. The OTPF also acknowledges that some of the values of the profession of occupational therapy are determined by cultural beliefs, including independence and roles (AOTA, 2008). Some of these values may differ from the values of clients and should be considered when engaging in practice (Iwama, 2004).

Student Activity: Defining Culture

Draft your personal definition of *culture*. Place your definition on an index card and hold on to it. View it at the conclusion of your lessons about culture to see how it has changed.

CULTURE-RELATED TERMINOLOGY

Culture presents a unique challenge to occupational therapy practitioners. According to Iwama (2004), "culture, in both common social and occupational therapy contexts, remains a slippery construct, taking on a variety of definitions and meanings depending on how it has been socially situated and by whom" (p. 1). Culture has many nuances that impact what people believe and understand about cultures. Defining these terms helps in understanding the dynamics of culture and why it is difficult to understand.

Diversity means a difference or variety that becomes exposed in human relationships (Gerstandt, 2007). Cultural diversity can lead to significant challenges in healthcare interactions, yet diversity is also what makes each individual pursue unique occupations. According to the Joint Position on Diversity published by the Canadian Association of Occupational Therapists (2007), no clear definition of diversity exists and commonly "diversity and cultural difference are often treated as if synonymous with ethnicity." Engaging in culturally sensitive practice embraces diversity, and learning about cultural diversity proves important in enhancing cultural awareness and critical self-reflection (Iwama, 2007; Murden, Norman, Ross, Sturdivant, Kedia, & Shah, 2008).

A *minority* is any group that is smaller than the majority. Minorities are often smaller groups of people with commonalities different from the majority. Minority groups are socially constructed and are generally, but not always, underserved (Tseng & Streltzer, 2008). However, minority groups usually have unique occupations that drive health beliefs, and research has shown that minorities do not feel these occupations are well understood by occupational therapy practitioners (Kirsh, Trentham, & Cole, 2006).

Ethnicity describes the "shared origins and shared culture" of a group (Loustanunau & Sobo, 1997, p. 28). Members of an ethnic group identify themselves collectively by a common history and a common set of behaviors. Ethnicity is not biologically based, and it does not infer culture. Common characteristics of an ethnic group include race, language, dialect, religion, literature, music, and food preferences (Glazner, 2006).

Another term frequently associated with culture is *race*. All human beings make up one race—the human race. Race is not a cultural identifier, and, according to McGruder, "race has no biological reality; it is a social construction that permeates our history and culture" (2007, presentation). Furthermore, race is "an unscientific, socially constructed taxonomy that is fluid and without boundaries" (Black & Wells, 2007, p. 342). Actually, more biological differences exist among people labeled in a certain "race" than similarities. When race is used to define risky behaviors or health predispositions, an ethical conundrum arises and a risk for racism occurs (Black & Wells, 2007). According to the Anti-Defamation League (2001), "racism is the belief that a particular race is superior or inferior to another, that a person's social and moral traits are predetermined by his or her inborn biological characteristics." Unfortunately, racism is still a prevalent and significant problem in health care and beyond (Kirsh, Trentham, & Cole, 2006).

The manifestations of racism are also important. People engage in racist and discriminatory acts based on bias, prejudice, and stereotype. A *bias* is simply a prejudice against another person, whereas *prejudice* means prejudgment of something or someone. Prejudices and biases can be based on many factors, including race, gender, ethnicity, religion, sexual preference, color of hair, or style (Black & Wells, 2007, p. 86). A *stereotype* is a generalization about a person or group of people (Black & Wells, 2007). Biases and prejudice can result from stereotypes. All three can lead to discrimination, which occurs when a person makes a decision based on differences or a bias, prejudice, or stereotype. *Discrimination* embodies an act towards a person based on a prejudice, bias, or stereotype and usually leads to problems in cross-cultural interactions (Black & Wells, 2007).

All of these terms are relevant and impact cross-cultural interactions on a daily basis. Furthermore, this terminology is crucial for students engaged in cross-cultural service-learning to not only know, but to understand. In order to strive for effective cross-cultural interactions, the student must be aware of his or her beliefs and how they enact each term described. Facing personal beliefs is never easy, and the challenge of recognizing personal biases, prejudices, and stereotypes can be difficult. However, facing personal beliefs is crucial to gaining cultural awareness and interacting in cross-cultural situations.

FACING OUR BELIEFS

Working in cross-cultural settings is challenging because it forces people to look inside themselves and face the personal biases and prejudices they hold against others. In cross-cultural service-learning activities, students will face firsthand personal biases, prejudices, and stereotypes. At times, these biases, prejudices, and stereotypes can lead to discrimination or disrupt a student's ability to engage in a service-learning activity appropriately. However, these challenges

Table 4-1 Lenses of Cultural Diversity.

Lens	Description
Assimilationist	Conform to the situation at hand.
Colorblind	Color is not an identifier.
Cultural centrist	Culture is central to personal identity.
Elitist	Membership in a specific group allows for special privileges.
Integrationist	Everyone should live in harmony despite differences.
Meritocratist	People who work hard and are of quality will succeed.
Multiculturalist	Embraces cultural diversity and desires more.
Seclusionist	Choose to engage in activities with similar people and believe this is important.
Transcendent	Believes in one human race.
Victim/Caretaker	People shall overcome injustices.

Sources: Abreu & Peloquin (2004), and Williams (2001).

can also be used as invaluable learning opportunities to teach these terms and how they impact healthcare interactions.

Although facing personal cultural beliefs presents a significant challenge to occupational therapy practitioners and students, acknowledging and discussing these beliefs is crucial to beginning a journey towards culturally competent practice. As discussed by Williams (2001) and applied to occupational therapy by Abreu and Peloquin (2004), people usually approach the world with their own lens for perceiving diversity (see Table 4-1). Based on this approach, occupational therapy practitioners and students view the world and their patients through a cultural lens that has been structured throughout personal life experiences.

Each practitioner or student engaging in cross-cultural interactions should take time to reflect upon their beliefs about diverse individuals. The lenses of cultural diversity provide a framework for reflecting on personal beliefs and how these manifest in cross-cultural interactions. When engaging students in service-learning in cross-cultural environments, reflection upon these factors will be crucial to ensure that students are able to provide appropriate cross-cultural interventions and learn about their personal cultural beliefs towards others.

Student Activity: Cultural Perception Essay

Based on the lenses listed in Table 4-1, which one do you identify most with? Write a one-page essay on why this lens fits you and how it will impact you as an occupational therapist. Discuss why you believe that you identify with that particular lens and whether it will be a strength or a challenge to you in practice.

CULTURAL COMPETENCE DEFINED

In an effort to address the diversity of the healthcare system, the drive for healthcare practitioners to attain cultural competence has become important (Black & Wells, 2007). In the healthcare professions, cultural competence has become important for the following reasons: to accommodate increasing diversity and demographic changes in United States; to address health disparities; to improve quality of care (Goode, 2003); to increase client compliance and satisfaction with therapy outcomes; to improve client satisfaction (Beach et al., 2005); and to adhere to professional, federal, and state requirements (Office of Minority Health, 2001). Cultural competence describes the ability to respond to the needs of a person or group of people from a culture other than one's own. According to Chiang and Carlson (2003), cultural competence "involves an awareness of one's own cultural beliefs and behaviors; cultural variables; health and disability issues relating to culture; and strategies for developing culturally sensitive practice" (p. 565). However, cultural competence is defined differently across the healthcare professions. Each healthcare discipline defines cultural competence uniquely

Table 4-2 Definitions of Cultural Competence by Profession.

Profession	Definition
Medicine	". . . process that requires individuals and healthcare systems to develop and expand their ability to effectively know about, be sensitive to, and have respect for cultural diversity" (AMSA, 2007).
Psychology	". . . possesses awareness of diversity, cultural knowledge, cross-cultural communication skills, and proper attitudes necessary to provide effective care for diverse populations" (APA, 2007).
Social work	". . . the process by which individuals and systems respond respectfully and effectively to people of all cultures, languages, classes, races, ethnic backgrounds, religions, and other diversity factors in a manner that recognizes, affirms, and values the worth of individuals, families, and communities and protects and preserves the dignity of each" (NASW, 2001, p. 11).
Physical therapy	"A set of congruent behaviors, attitudes, and policies that come together in a system, agency, or among professionals and enable that system, agency, or those professionals to work effectively in cross-cultural situations" (APTA, 2008).
Occupational therapy	"Cultural competency is a journey rather than an end. It refers to the process of actively developing and practicing appropriate, relevant, and sensitive strategies and skills in interacting with culturally different persons" (AOTA, 1995).

and educates its practitioners toward the chosen belief system (Table 4-2).

CULTURAL COMPETENCE THEORIES

The term *cultural competence* is a bit of misnomer, because no one person can be competent in all the cultures of the world, and it is questionable that anyone could ever be truly "competent" in a culture other than his or her own. Multiple theoretical approaches exist for attaining cultural competence in healthcare interactions. These theoretical approaches provide frameworks for healthcare professionals to strive for culturally competent practice. Not only are these models relevant to practice, but they can also be used to frame and teach culture using a service-learning pedagogical approach. Utilizing cultural competence theories in service learning can aid students in helping bridge gaps and apply the concepts of culture in a real-world setting.

The Purnell model of cultural competence comes out of nursing, but was meant for use in all the health professions. Physical therapy used this model as a basis for the book *Developing Cultural Competence in Physical Therapy Practice* (Lattanzi & Purnell, 2006). In the Purnell model, cultural competence is viewed as a nonlinear and conscious process by the healthcare professional (Purnell, 2002). The Purnell model for cultural competence "does not deal with the objective culture including arts, music, literature, and the humanities, but rather addresses the subjective culture of attitudes, beliefs, values, behaviors, and practices in the context of healthcare" (Lattanzi & Purnell, 2006, p. 26). Furthermore, the Purnell model guides "professionals in developing a broad understanding of culture and assist them in providing more culturally competent examinations, evaluations, prognoses, and interventions across a wide range of impairments, functional limitations and disabilities" (Purnell & Lattanzi, 2006, p. 27).

Purnell's model consists of 12 domains couched within the global society, community, family, and person. The 12 domains include heritage, communication, family roles and organization, workforce issues, biocultural ecology, high-risk behaviors, nutrition, pregnancy, death rituals, spirituality, healthcare practices, and healthcare practitioners. The model provides a holistic framework for understanding a client's culture and supplying intervention based on cultural views (Purnell, 2002).

In Purnell's model, cultural competence is viewed on a continuum; healthcare providers range on a continuum of cultural competence from unconsciously incompetent to unconsciously competent. An unconsciously incompetent healthcare provider is one who acts in a culturally insensitive manner, but does not know he or she is acting in a culturally insensitive manner. A consciously incompetent healthcare provider represents an individual who knowingly acts in a culturally insensitive manner and may exhibit racist and biased behaviors. A consciously competent provider is a person who knowingly makes an active effort to act in a culturally sensitive manner. Finally, the unconsciously competent provider represents an individual who unknowingly acts in a culturally sensitive manner and acting in this manner is second nature (Purnell, 2002).

Another cultural competence model from the nursing literature that applies to all healthcare professionals is the process of cultural competence in the delivery of healthcare services, created by Campinha-Bacote (2002; 2005). In this model, cultural competence is viewed through the metaphor of a volcano and described as "the process in which the healthcare provider continuously strives to achieve the ability to effectively work within the cultural context of a client, individual, family or community" (Campinha-Bacote, 2001, p. 8; see Table 4-3). The foundation of the volcano is cultural desire,

Table 4-3 Concepts of Cultural Competence in the Campinha-Bacote Model.

Concept	Description
Cultural desire	A desire to engage in seeking cultural competence
Cultural awareness	Develop respect, appreciation, and sensitivity to values, beliefs, etc. Self-exploration
Cultural humility	Lifelong commitment to personal self-reflection
Cultural knowledge	Seeking and educating oneself on culture Understanding worldviews
Cultural encounters	Engaging in cross-cultural experiences
Cultural skill	Ability to collect cultural data Assess clients in a culturally appropriate manner

Sources: Campinha-Bacote (1998; 2002).

which is the desire to engage in seeking cultural competence. In this model, healthcare professionals must have a desire for learning about the culture, because without it, all the other steps in attaining cultural competence are irrelevant. Cultural desire permeates the volcano allowing the healthcare provider to make decisions through attaining cultural awareness, cultural humility, cultural knowledge, and cultural skill.

The Cross model of cultural competency (1988; 1989), a model out of social work, provides a continuum for healthcare providers to follow in attaining cultural competence. According to Cross (1988), cultural competence "is a set of congruent behaviors, attitudes and policies that come together in a system, agency or professional and enable that system, agency or professional to work effectively in cross-cultural situations." In this model, cultural competence is attained through a developmental sequence on a continuum, including cultural destructiveness, cultural incapacity, cultural blindness, cultural precompetence, cultural competence, and cultural proficiency (Table 4-4).

Arthur Kleinman (1978), a physician and medical anthropologist, developed the explanatory model of illness, which incorporates eight questions to gather a patient's perspective on his or her illness. The purpose of the explanatory model is to explore the patient's perspective, which is a valuable aspect of cross-cultural interactions as well as client-centered occupational therapy practice. These questions, located in Table 4-5, can be used during patient interviews to explore a patient's health beliefs and views on the source of the illness. Because culture drives many health beliefs about disease and illness, the explanatory model is essential to cross-cultural practice.

Student Activity: Cross-Cultural Interview

Conduct an interview with a community member. Use the questions from the explanatory model of illness to explore the health beliefs of this individual.

Table 4-4 Development Stages of Cross Model of Cultural Competency.

Stage	Description
Cultural destructiveness	• Attitudes and practices destructive to cultures and to the individuals in the culture • Actively enforce racist policies or advocate for differential treatment of groups of individuals based on culture
Cultural incapacity	• Not intentionally seeking to be culturally destructive • Lack the capacity to help minority clients • Believing in racial superiority of the dominant group
Cultural blindness	• Believing that culture/ethnicity/race make no difference in how services are provided • Believe approaches traditionally used by dominant culture are universally applicable • People in this stage often claim color-blindness
Cultural precompetence	• Individuals realize weaknesses in serving minorities • Attempt to improve aspects of their services to a specific population by learning specific information about culture's health practices
Cultural competence	• Accepting and respecting differences • Continual self-assessment • Learn specific cultural information integrate this information into patient care
Cultural proficiency	• Hold other cultures in high • Influence institutional policies, procedures, and protocols to advocate for quality patient care

Source: Cross (1988).

Table 4-5 Explanatory Model of Illness Questions.

- What do you call your problem? What name does it have?
- What do you think caused your problem?
- Why do you think it started when it did?
- What does your sickness do to you? How does it work?
- How severe is it? Will it have a short or long course?
- What do you fear most about your disorder?
- What are the chief problems that your sickness has caused for you?
- What kind of treatment do you think you should receive?
- What are the most important results you hope to receive from the treatment?

Source: Kleinman et al. (1978).

Across the healthcare literature, cultural competence and the best approaches for attaining cultural competence have been the topics of much discussion. Service-learning has been proposed and evidenced as a model to enhance cultural competence for students in the health professions (Flannery & Ward, 1999; Nokes, Nickitas, Keida, & Neville, 2005; Burnett, Hamel, & Long, 2004).

CULTURE AND SERVICE-LEARNING

As a pedagogical model, service-learning provides real-world experience and can be invaluable in areas difficult to simulate in a classroom (Rubin, 2004). It allows students to experience "greater breadth and depth of experience by involving them in social, political, cultural, environmental, and other important aspects" of a community (Burnett, Hamel, & Long, 2004, p. 181). The dynamics of culture and its influences on healthcare interactions can be discussed at length, but true learning occurs when students face the challenges of such interactions. Furthermore, service-learning has proven student outcomes of deeper understanding of social issues, enhanced lifelong learning, and improved problem-solving and reasoning skills to address complex social problems (Eyler, 2002). These are tied directly to the skills necessary for becoming a culturally competent practitioner, presenting a valid reason for using service-learning as a method for teaching cross-cultural skills. In a review of interventions used by academicians teaching cultural competence, 11 used cultural immersion as a method for teaching cultural competence to health professions students (Beach et al., 2005).

In the literature, it has been demonstrated that students who engage in service-learning are able to interact with those different than themselves, a key skill in cross-cultural interactions (Hanks, 2003; Clark, 2000). Rubin (2004) identified that dental students immersed in the community learned both compassion and empathy towards diverse individuals. Interestingly, Nokes and colleagues (2005) found that service-learning activities did not increase cultural competence among nursing students. However, students ranked themselves very highly on pretests of cultural competence and much lower on posttests after service-learning experiences, indicating a realization of the lack of cultural competence and the challenges of cross-cultural interactions (Nokes et al., 2005). The literature demonstrates a track record of success across the health professions in the use of service-learning as a viable approach to teaching the concepts of cultural competence in a rich, authentic environment.

Student Activity: Global Store Exploration

One of the most accessible ways to learn about another culture is through food. Go to a local global store in your community and pick out a global food item that is unfamiliar to you. Do research to find out more about the food item and its cultural meanings through reading, interviewing, asking questions, or other appropriate means. Form small groups and share your item and what you learned with your peers.

DEVELOPING CROSS-CULTURAL SKILLS FOR CROSS-CULTURAL SERVICE-LEARNING

Developing cross-cultural skills is not an easy or quick process. However, key skills exist that can aid occupational therapy students and practitioners in cross-cultural environments. Being aware of these skills is a crucial first step prior to engaging in a cultural service-learning activity.

The following skills are crucial to cross-cultural interactions:

1. **Cultural self-assessment.** Across the cultural-competence literature, the first step in developing cross-cultural skills is engaging in a cultural self-assessment to gain perspectives into personal cultural self-awareness (Black & Wells, 2007). In this process, the individual explores their worldview, exploring personal cultural beliefs and values. Through this exploration, the student needs to reflect upon personal beliefs about others, including personal views about individuals from diverse cultures. Critical self-reflection is not only necessary at the beginning of a journey towards cultural competence, but throughout a professional career. Reflection allows for an exploration of the rights and wrongs of a situation in order to prepare for the next similar experience. Furthermore, awareness of beliefs and values allows the student to explore how personal beliefs and values will impact clinical reasoning and future patient interactions.

   Self-assessment should be done prior to engagement in cross-cultural service learning to prepare students for community experiences. Students will go into communities with at least the knowledge and recognition of the importance of understanding the perspectives of others. Furthermore, an initial assessment sets the tone for engaging students in ongoing reflective activities. See the student activity for an outline of a self-assessment to be used to explore cultural views.

2. **Acknowledge lack of knowledge.** No healthcare provider could possibly ever know all the cultural knowledge needed to interact with their diverse clientele. However, it is important to be able to acknowledge a lack of knowledge and to move forward to attain that knowledge for the best patient outcomes (Brach & Fraserirector, 2000). A culturally competent practitioner must always be willing to seek information about a diverse client. Appropriate approaches include asking questions, reading about the culture, observing the culture, cross-cultural

---

Student Activity: Cultural Self-Assessment

Answer the following questions to engage in cultural self-assessment.
 Analyze your values:

1. Am I sensitive to others who are different than me?
2. What is meaningful to me from my culture?
3. How does what is meaningful to me influence my health beliefs?
4. Do I have biases, prejudices, or stereotypes against others?
5. If so, where do they come from?

Evaluate your self-concept with other cultures:

6. Do I feel comfortable around those who are different than me?
7. If you feel comfortable, why?

---

training, community immersion, and engaging in cultural activities (Glazner, 2006). All of these activities can take place during a service-learning experience and should be included to enhance the cross-cultural learning.

3. **Develop and practice communication skills.** Awareness of communication, including both verbal and nonverbal communication, is crucial to interacting with diverse clients. In any cross-cultural interaction, communication is a crucial to building rapport and sustaining a relationship. Miscommunication can lead to healthcare errors impacting client outcomes and damaging a patient's trust in healthcare professionals (Safeer & Keenan, 2005).

Language is impacted by word choice, linguistics, and voice, which are all culturally driven. In cross-cultural communication, students need to be aware of multiple factors, including culturally appropriate language; awareness of nonverbal communication, both of the client and the student; health literacy and Culturally and Linguistically Appropriate Services (CLAS). In cross-cultural communication, it is crucial to be aware of terms and gestures that indicate disrespect. These vary based on the client's culture and should be explored prior to engagement.

Health literacy is also important to cross-cultural communication. According to Healthy People 2010, *health literacy* is defined as "the degree to which individuals have the capacity to obtain, process, and understand basic health information and services needed to make appropriate health decisions" (U.S. Department of Health and Human Services, 2000, p. 11-4). Health literacy is not simply the ability to read health information, but also the ability to have conversations with healthcare professionals and to navigate and make healthcare decisions (Glassman, 2008). Occupational therapy students and practitioners need to be knowledgeable about a patient's health literacy level in order to provide proper instructions, health education, and home exercise plans, along with teaching the activities of daily living, such as medication management.

CLAS provides a framework for healthcare providers to respond to patients' cultural and language needs (Office of Minority Health, 2001). The goals of CLAS are to address healthcare inequities, to provide fair and equal treatment, to address language barriers between healthcare providers and patients, and to increase the ability of healthcare providers to respond to the needs of diverse patients (Table 4-6). CLAS provides a common language for discussing the challenges of cross-cultural practice.

Service-learning provides an opportunity to practice cross-cultural communication (Brown & Howard, 2005). Students have opportunities to practice communication skills in cross-cultural settings where the stakes may not be as high as in a healthcare situation. Improving cross-cultural communication can aid students in preparation for future clinical interactions (Buchanan & Witlen, 2006). Furthermore, students gain a consciousness of the challenges of communication and how it can either empower or disempower healthcare clients (Crabtree, 1998).

Table 4–6 Culturally and Linguistically Appropriate Services (CLAS).

Standard 1: Provide effective, understandable, and respectful care in a manner compatible with cultural health beliefs and preferred language.

Standard 2: Implement strategies to recruit, retain, and promote a diverse staff and leadership.

Standard 3: Ensure that staff at all levels and across all disciplines receive ongoing education and training in CLAS service delivery.

Standard 4: Offer and provide language assistance (e.g., bilingual staff and interpreters).

Standard 5: Inform patients orally and in writing of their right to receive language assistance.

Standard 6: Assure the competence of language assistance provided. Family and friends should not be used to interpret.

Standard 7: Make available materials and post signage in commonly used languages.

Standard 8: Develop, implement, and promote a written strategic plan to provide CLAS services.

Standard 9: Conduct ongoing organizational self-assessments of CLAS activities.

Standard 10: Collect data on patients' race, ethnicity, and spoken and written language.

Standard 11: Maintain a current demographic, cultural, and epidemiological profile of the community and conduct needs assessment.

Standard 12: Develop collaborative partnerships with communities. Facilitate community/patient involvement.

Standard 13: Provide culturally sensitive conflict and grievance resolution processes.

Standard 14: Make public information about the organization's progress in implementing the CLAS standards.

Source: Office of Minority Health (2001).

4. **Recognize professional power.** Health beliefs of cultural groups do not only apply to health issues, but also to relationships with healthcare providers. In many cultures, healthcare providers are viewed as powerful authority figures to be obeyed and whose advice is to be followed (Black & Wells, 2007). In most healthcare interactions, the healthcare provider is in

---

Student Activity: CLAS Application

For each CLAS standard, brainstorm the role for occupational therapy practitioners in culturally appropriate care.

---

power with knowledge and information to provide to patients, often entitled professional power. Healthcare providers possess a professional title that promotes expectations of power and knowledge.

Power plays a role in culture and can lead to oppression. Service-learning provides pedagogy for teaching the importance of recognizing professional power (Pompa, 2002). Students are given the opportunity to explore oppression and the power of working with the underserved in a community context (Deans, 1999). Reflection and class discussions can be geared towards exploring the concept of power. Classroom activities to explore power and powerlessness are located in the student activity entitled The Blind Walk.

5. **Learn health beliefs.** Health beliefs are basically just beliefs about health that are based on culture. The origins and beliefs about illness and how it occurs are often based in a person's

---

Student Activity: The Blind Walk

Choose a partner. One partner is blindfolded. The other partner leads the blindfolded partner to the bathroom to wash his or her hands. When this activity has been completed, discuss the following reflection questions:

1. How did it feel to be totally dependent on another person?
2. How did it feel to be in control of another person to lead them wherever you want?
3. What are the dynamics of power and powerlessness here?
4. How could these themes play out in community situations? In healthcare interactions?

cultural beliefs. Health beliefs determine what people believe about food, body image, caregiving, pain, stress, and health care in general.

If interacting in a healthcare context for service-learning, the occupational therapy students should be aware of some basic health beliefs of the people with whom they will interact in order to promote appropriate cultural interactions. However, students should also be prepared to learn and reflect on these beliefs that may be significantly different from their own. These may include factors such as the beliefs about healthy foods and exercise. For example, in the case that a food is very important to the culture, students should not deem it unhealthy without understanding the food's importance. Approaches to health education should be focused on the health beliefs of the cultural group (Lockhart & Resick, 1997).

6. **Engage in active reflection.** Reflection is key to the application and processing of knowledge in service-learning pedagogy. Reflection has long been studied since its introduction by Dewey (Dewey, 1933; Rodgers, 2002) and further studied by experts such as Kolb (1984). Reflection is a valuable teaching tool, helping students "develop the capacity for critical thought if they are challenged both by surprising experiences and by reflective teachers who help them explore these experiences and question their fundamental assumptions about their world" (Eyler, 2002, p. 521).

Research in service-learning has demonstrated that service-learning experiences with high levels of reflection promote students' abilities to problem-solve complex issues (Eyler, 2002). But reflection is not automatic and needs to be constructed for students in a way that challenges them to engage in critical thought processes (Eyler, 2002). Eyler argued that in order for reflection to be effective in impacting cognitive development in students, it has to be rich and occur at multiple levels. Students should reflect individually, in small groups and with community partners on a continuum from prior to the service, during service experiences and after the service experience.

Table 4-7 Types of Active Reflection.

- Reflection on cultural self-assessment
- Cultural strategic plan—a set of goals and objectives for attaining culturally appropriate skills
- Journaling
- Group discussion
- Online discussion boards
- Blogging
- Artistic expression—skits, collages, drawings, paintings, etc.
- Community assessment
- Community discussion

Source: Eyler (2002).

Multiple methods for engaging students in active reflection related to service-learning exist (Eyler, 2002). Table 4-7 outlines types of active reflection beneficial for cross-cultural interactions. When analyzing culture in a service-learning experience, students have the opportunities to reflect upon many factors, including focusing on development of cross-cultural skills and the challenges of working in a cross-cultural environment. Furthermore, students can focus on the complex health issues that impact the cultural group. Many of the aspects discussed in this section, including professional power, communication, and health beliefs, can be foundations for reflection.

THE COMMUNITY AS A CULTURAL CLASSROOM: BEST PRACTICES FOR EDUCATORS

The community can provide a forum for learning the concepts of culture and how occupational therapy students can provide culturally appropriate care. Service-learning provides a pedagogy for teaching culturally appropriate care by providing students with real-world experiences. Students can be immersed in a community that is culturally diverse and engage in activities that challenge cultural beliefs and develop cross-cultural skills.

Best practices identify how to be successful in teaching culturally appropriate skills using a service-learning approach. Many of these best practices align with general best practices for service-learning. Yet, it is important to reiterate these best practices in the context of cross-cultural service learning.

1. **Develop community-driven activities.** All community-based service-learning should be centered on the community, exploring both the community's needs and assets (Kretzmann & McKnight, 1993). In a cultural context, this concept is especially important. Cultural groups face many challenges in the healthcare arena, such as feelings of discrimination and a lack of respect from healthcare providers (Kirsh, Trentham, & Cole, 2006). Developing service-learning activities with the community and culture in mind will help decrease feelings of discrimination and promote community buy-in to the partnership.

2. **Promote student buy-in.** In order for students to learn, they, themselves, have to find value in the service-learning experience. A best practice for this is to empower students with a choice and promote passion for a community partner. A strategy to aid in this process is to invite community partner representatives to a class period to share the mission of the organization and to describe the people they serve. When community members tell their stories, the students are provided with an authentic context, which prepares them for experiences in and with the community. Furthermore, this process alleviates anxiety, which is common when being asked to explore an unknown community.

   After listening to the community members, students are asked to draft a persuasive essay identifying which community partner best suits their learning objectives and whom they have a passion to serve. Appendix A contains the Community Partner Justification Assignment which requires students to identify the community partner of their choice. Students will be matched based on preferences and the persuasiveness of the essay. This activity not only encourages passion and active reflection, but begins to put a face to the community, building the passion to serve that ultimately promotes lifelong service (Eyler, 2002).

3. **Tie service to learning objectives.** Besides buying-in to the community and building a passion to serve, students need to clearly understand how service-learning is tied to the course's culture-related learning objectives (Begley, Doll, & Ryan-Haddad, 2008). Reflection can be framed around these learning objectives, and reiterating them in class discussions is important. Students need to know why they are engaged in service-learning and the purposes for learning outcomes in order to be successful (Eyler, 2002).

   In the context of learning cross-cultural skills, learning objectives can be clearly tied to the experience. Examples include practicing cross-cultural communication, analysis of cultural competence theories, and reflection on complex cultural health beliefs that impact the patient–practitioner relationship. Whatever the goals and purpose of the course, service-learning provides students a forum to engage in cross-cultural interactions and practice cross-cultural skills. Learning objectives related directly to culture-related course material easily translates into community experiences as long as students' expectations are clearly articulated.

4. **Engage students in active reflection.** As discussed previously, active reflection is important to service-learning pedagogy (Eyler, 2002). Reflection needs to occur before, during, and after the experience. Cross-cultural experiences challenge students, forcing them to face personal issues in diverse environments. Reflection questions need to be sensitive to these factors, and the instructor needs to react to the reflections appropriately. For example, in an occupational therapy culture course, several students in individual reflections expressed a concern for personal safety when going to a community partner site. In order to address the concerns, students developed a group protocol for

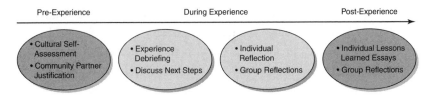

Figure 4-1 Best practice reflection continuum for cross-cultural service-learning.

safety in the community that each member agreed upon. This protocol was also communicated to the community partner site and all agreed to comply. In later reflections, fears were alleviated and students were able to move on to focus on learning objectives. Appendix B offers a wide variety of reflection questions beneficial for cross-cultural service learning (D. Palowski, September 2009, personal communication).

CONCLUSION

The dynamics of culture are complex and difficult to teach to occupational therapy students. However, service-learning provides a pedagogical approach for promoting students' exposure to diverse patients and for practicing the cross-cultural skills necessary for being an effective occupational therapy practitioner. This chapter presented a foundation for both students and educators exploring cross-cultural service-learning. Service-learning, in itself, is challenging and adding the dynamics of culture adds further complication. However, the opportunity to explore the complexity of cross-cultural interactions in an authentic context is an invaluable student learning experience.

REFERENCES

Abreu, B. C., & Peloquin, S. M. (2004). The issue is: Embracing diversity in our profession. *American Journal of Occupational Therapy, 58*(3), 353–359.
American Medical Student Association (AMSA). (2007). Cultural competency in medicine. Retrieved November 26, 2007, from http://www.amsa.org/programs/gpit/cultural.cfm.

American Occupational Therapy Association (AOTA). (2008). Occupational therapy practice framework: Domain and process, 2nd edition. *American Journal of Occupational Therapy, 62*(6), 625–683.

American Occupational Therapy Association, Multicultural Task Force. (1995). Definition and terms. Bethesda, MD: American Occupational Therapy Association.

American Physical Therapy Association (APTA). (2008). Tips to increase cultural competency. Retrieved December 2, 2008, from http://www.apta.org/AM/Template.cfm?Section=Cultural_Competence1&Template=/TaggedPage/TaggedPageDisplay.cfm&TPLID=48&ContentID=20219.

American Psychological Association (APA). (2007). Cultural competence. Retrieved October 15, 2009, from http://www.apa.org/.

Anti-Defamation League. (2001). Racism. Retrieved September 1, 2009, from http://www.adl.org/hate-patrol/racism.asp.

Beach, M. C., Price, E. G., Gary, T. L., Robinson, K. A., Gozu, A., Palacio, A., et al. (2005). Cultural competence: A systematic review of healthcare provider educational interventions. *Medical Care, 43*(4), 356–373.

Begley, K., Doll, J. D., & Ryan-Haddad, A. (2008). Putting the pieces together: Building scholarship around community engagement for health professions students. Office of Faculty Development Presentation, Omaha, Nebraska, April 2008.

Black, R. M., & Wells, S. A. (2007). *Culture and occupation.* Bethesda, MD: AOTA Press.

Bonder, B., Martin, L., & Miracle, A. (2002). *Culture in clinical care.* Thorofare, NJ: Slack.

Brach, C., & Fraserirector, I. (2000). Can cultural competency reduce racial and ethnic health disparities? A review and conceptual model. *Medical Care Research and Review, 57*(1), 181–217.

Brown, E. L., & Howard, B. R. (2005). Becoming culturally responsive teachers through service-learning: A case study of five novice teachers. *Multicultural Education, 12*(4), 2–4.

Buchanan, D., & Witlen, R. (2006). Balancing service and education: Ethical management of student-run clinics. *Journal of Health Care for the Poor and Underserved, 17*(3), 477–485.

Burnett, J. D., Hamel, D., & Long, L. L. (2004). Service learning in graduate counseling education: Developing multicultural counseling competency. *Journal of Multicultural Counseling and Development, 32*, 180–191.

Campinha-Bacote, J. (2005). A culturally conscious approach to holistic nursing. Program and abstracts of the American Holistic Nurses Association Conference, June 16–19, 2005, King of Prussia, Pennsylvania.

Campinha-Bacote, J. (2002). The process of cultural competence in the delivery of healthcare services: A model of care. *Journal of Transcultural Nursing, 13*, 181–184.

Campinha-Bacote, J. (2001). A model of practice to address cultural competence in rehabilitation nursing. *Rehabilitation Nursing, 26*(1), 8–11.

Campinha-Bacote, J. (1998). *The process of cultural competence in the delivery of healthcare services,* 4th ed. Cincinnati, OH: Transcultural C.A.R.E. Associates.

Canadian Association of Occupational Therapists. (2007). Joint position on diversity. Retrieved December 8, 2008, from http://www.caot.ca/default.asp?pageID=2120.

Chiang, M., & Carlson, G. (2003). Occupational therapy in multicultural contexts: Issues and strategies. *British Journal of Occupational Therapy, 66*(12), 559–567.

Clark, G. (2000). Messages from Josefa: Service learning in Mexico. *Language and Learning Across the Disciplines, 4*(3), 76–80.

Crabtree, R. D. (1998). Mutual empowerment in cross-cultural participatory development and service learning: Lessons in communication and social justice from projects in El Salvador and Nicaragua. *Journal of Applied Communication Research, 26,* 182–209.

Cross, T. L., Bazron, B., Dennis, K., & Isaacs, M. (1989). Toward a culturally competent system of care. Available from CAASP Technical Assistance Center, Georgetown University Child Development Center, 3800 Reservoir Rd., NW, Washington, DC, 20007.

Cross, T. (1988). Cultural competence continuum. Retrieved December 3, 2008, from http://www.nysccc.org/T-Rarts/Articles/CultCompCont.html.

Deans, T. (1999). Service learning in two keys: Paulo Freire's critical pedagogy in relation to John Dewey's pragmatism. *Michigan Journal of Community Service Learning, 6,* 15–29.

Dewey, J. (1933). *How we think: A restatement of the relation of reflective thinking to the educative process.* Boston: D.C. Heath.

Eyler, J. (2002). Reflection: Linking service and learning—linking students and communities. *Journal of Social Issues, 58*(3), 517–534.

Flannery, D., & Ward, K. (1999). Service learning: A vehicle for developing cultural competence in health education. *American Journal of Health Behavior, 23*(5), 323–331.

Gerstandt, J. (2007). Working with humans. Presented at Diversity Workshop, Omaha, Nebraska.

Glassman, P. (2008). Health literacy. Retrieved October 7, 2008, from http://nnlm.gov/outreach/consumer/hlthlit.html#A1.

Glazner, L. K. (2006). Cultural diversity for health professions. *Work, 26,* 297–302.

Goode, T. D., Sockalingam, S., Bronheim, S., Brown, M., & Jones, W. (2003). A planner's guide—infusing principles, content and themes related to cultural and linguistic competence into meetingsand conferences. Retrieved October 23, 2009, from www11.georgetown.edu/research/gucchd/nccc/documents/Planners_Guide.pdf.

Hanks, C. (2003). Health disparities research and service learning. *Journal of Multicultural Nursing and Health, 9,* 18–23. Retrieved December 2, 2008, from http://findarticles.com/p/articles/mi_qa3919/is_200310/ai_n9309684.

Helman, C. G. (2001). *Culture, health and illness.* London: Arnold Publishers.

Iwama, M. K. (2007). Embracing diversity: Explaining the cultural dimensions of our occupational therapeutic selves. *New Zealand Journal of Occupational Therapy, 54*(2), 16–23.

Iwama, M. K. (2004). Meaning and inclusion: Revisiting culture in occupational therapy. *Australian Journal of Occupational Therapy, 51,* 1–2.

Kleinman, A., Eisenberg, L., & Good, B. (1978). Culture, illness and care: Clinical lessons from anthropologic and cross-cultural research. *Annals of Internal Medicine, 88,* 251–258.

Kirsh, B., Trentham, B., & Cole, S. (2006). Diversity in occupational therapy: Experiences of consumers who identify themselves as minority member groups. *Australian Occupational Therapy Journal, 53,* 302–313.

Kolb, D. (1984). *Experiential learning: Experience as the source of learning and development.* Englewood Cliffs, NJ: Prentice Hall.

Kretzmann, J. P., & McKnight, J. L. (1993). *Building communities from the inside out: A path toward finding and mobilizing a community's assets.* Skokie, IL: ACTA Publications.

Lattanzi, J. B., & Purnell, L. D. (2006). *Developing cultural competence in physical therapy practice.* Philadelphia, PA: F.A. Davis.

Lockhart, J. S., & Resick, L.K. (1997). Teaching cultural competence: The value of experiential learning and community resources. *Nurse Educator, 22*(3), 27–31.

Loustanunau, M. O., & Sobo, E. J. (1997). *The Cultural Context of Health, Illness and Medicine.* London: Bergin & Garvey.

McGruder, J. (2007). *Sociocultural Awareness Workshop.* Presented at the American Occupational Therapy Association Conference, St. Louis, Missouri. April 2007.

Mish, F. (Ed.). (2008). *Merriam Webster Online Dictionary.* Retrieved December 9, 2008, from http://www.merriam-webster.com/dictionary/culture.

Murden, R., Norman, A., Ross, J., Sturdivant, E., Kedia, M., & Shah, S. (2008). Occupational therapy students' perceptions of their cultural awareness and competence. *Occupational Therapy International, 15*(3), 191–203.

National Association for Social Workers (NASW). (2001). NASW Standards for Cultural Competence in social work practice. Retrieved December 2, 2008, from http://www.socialworkers.org/practice/standards/NASWCultural Standards.pdf.

Nokes, K. M., Nickitas, D. M., Keida, R., & Neville, S. (2005). Does service learning increase cultural competency, critical thinking, and civic engagement. *Journal of Nursing Education, 44*(2), 65–70.

Office of Minority Health. (2001). *National Standards for Culturally and Linguistically Appropriate Services in Health Care: Final Report.* Washington, DC: U.S. Department of Health and Human Services.

Pompa, L. (2002). Service learning as crucible: Reflections on immersion, context, power, and transformation. *Michigan Journal of Community Service Learning, 9*(1), 67–76.

Purnell, L. (2002). The Purnell model for cultural competence. *Journal of Transcultural Nursing, 13*(3), 193–196.

Rodgers, C. (2002). Defining reflection: Another look at John Dewey and reflective thinking. *The Teachers College Record, 104*(4), 842–866.

Rubin, R. W. (2004). Developing cultural competence and social responsibility in preclinical dental students. *Journal of Dental Education, 68*(4), 460–467.

Rudman, D. L., & Dennhardt, S. (2008). Shaping knowledge regarding occupation: Examining the cultural underpinnings of the evolving concept of occupational identity. *Australian Journal of Occupational Therapy, 55*, 153–162.

Safeer, R. S., & Keenan, J. (2005). Health literacy: The gap between physicians and patients. *American Family Physician, 72*(3), 387–388.

Spector, R. E. (2004). *Cultural diversity in health and illness,* 6th ed. Upper Saddle River, NJ: Prentice Hall.

Tseng, W. S., & Streltzer, J. (2008). *Cultural competence in health care.* New York: Springer.

U.S. Department of Health and Human Services. (2000). *Healthy People 2010: Understanding and Improving Health,* 2nd ed. Washington, DC: U.S. Government Printing Office.

Wilcock, A. (2006). *An Occupational Perspective on Health* (2nd Ed.). Thorofare, NJ: Slack.

Williams, M. (2001). *The 10 lenses: Your guide to living & working in a multicultural world.* Herndon, VA: Capital Books.

Community Partner Justification Assignment

Student Name: _____

Top Choice: _____

2nd Choice: _____

3rd Choice: _____

No Preference (put an X): _____

Why did you choose your top choice?

What are your learning objectives for this experience related to the course? (Write at least 3)

What community partner would you least like? Why?

If you have no preference, why?

Sample Reflection Questions

1. What were your first impressions of your community partner?
2. What questions/concerns do you have in working with this partner?
3. What do you see as the strengths/positives in working with this partner?
4. What is one thing you already learned from your partner?
5. What did you do with your service partner the last time you met with him/her? What things did you talk about?
6. Thus far, do you feel successful, effective in what you wanted to accomplish?
7. How are you applying the concepts from class into your experiential learning?
8. How has this experience enhanced your personally?
9. What is it that is frustrating or challenging about this experience?
10. Think about your experiences throughout the semester with your community partner. If you were to identify a metaphor/

simile that describes your experiences with this service-learning project, what would it be?

My community partner and/or my learning experience is or is like _____

Provide a diagram/picture of your metaphor and in a one-page description of linking your metaphor with your experiences and your text; explain your choice. In doing so, use three text ideas (clearly identifying with page numbers) in your rationale.

Logistics: One-page – typed.

Source: Modified from Donna Palowsky.

Chapter 5

Providing Voice to Vulnerable Populations Through Service-Learning Infused in an Occupational Therapy Program

Ingrid M. Provident, EdD, OTR/L
Anne Marie Witchger Hansen, MS, OTR/L
Jaime Phillip Muñoz, PhD, OTR, FAOTA

Service-learning, as pedagogy for occupational therapy education, parallels the philosophical and theoretical teachings of Dewey (1938) and Boyer's (1994) call for "engaged citizenry," connecting the rich resources of the university to our most pressing social, civic, and ethical problems, as a primary mission and purpose of American higher education. This pedagogy embodies a social vision of occupational therapy that advocates for the profession to fully embrace our moral responsibility to address the significant social injustices that exist in our communities (Kronenberg, Algado, & Pollard, 2005; Townsend, 1993; Watson & Swartz, 2004).

This social vision of occupational therapy is grounded in a central value of the profession: to honor and promote the dignity and worth of every person (Kielhofner, 2004). The centrality of the profession's emphasis on human dignity permeates a number of official documents, which explicitly articulate this value; for example, the Occupational Therapy Code of Ethics (2005), Core Values and Attitudes of Occupational Therapy Practice (AOTA, 1993), The Philosophical Base of Occupational Therapy (AOTA, 1995), and the Occupational Therapy Practice Framework: Domain and Process (AOTA, 2002). These documents delineate the core values of our profession and emphasize enablement, empowerment, and participation. They also represent a call to address pressing societal issues through processes that promote collaboration. Honoring human dignity through service is also a foundational principle of authentic service-learning experiences (Bickford & Reynolds, 2002; Cuban & Anderson, 2007; Rimmerman, 1997; Wade, 2001; Westheimer & Kahne, 2004).

A primary objective of service-learning is to extend academic learning through engagement in authentic community service (McGowan, 2002). Community-based service-learning opportunities provide students with a natural context for broadening their understanding of community health and healthcare systems, multiculturalism, and occupational and social justice (Witchger Hansen et al., 2007). Learning from people whose daily patterns of occupational functioning are influenced by poverty, limited resources, marginalization, and stigmatization can help students appreciate the lived experience of health disparities (Kronenberg, Algado, & Pollard, 2005; Muñoz, 2007; Townsend, 1993; Townsend & Whiteford, 2005). When structured guided reflection is employed, students can also learn the processes whereby they may become effective "health agents" (Yerxa, 1983) who work toward reducing social injustices in their own communities (Hatcher, Bringle, & Muthiah, 2004).

This chapter provides a brief history of the development of service-learning in the Department of Occupational Therapy at Duquesne University. First, we will describe the evolution of our efforts to craft service-learning opportunities that target the healthcare needs of vulnerable populations. Second, we will identify the processes we used to facilitate the development of behaviors and attitudes that support professionalism and practice scholarship. Third, we will delineate the processes used to develop and sustain effective, reciprocal community–university partnerships and the methods we employed to generate service-learning opportunities at a variety of community sites. Finally, specific descriptions of courses, learning activities, guided reflection exercises, course evaluations, and community outcome measures will be presented to exemplify the processes used.

INSTITUTIONAL CONTEXT: EDUCATION FOR THE MIND, HEART, AND SOUL

Since its inception in 1994, the curriculum of the occupational therapy program at Duquesne University in Pittsburgh, Pennsylvania, has infused principles of service-learning throughout the curriculum and has intentionally coordinated courses to provide a sequenced and incrementally challenging set of community-based experiential teaching/learning activities.

Service-learning at Duquesne University's occupational therapy department is influenced by the institutional context, specifically by its identity as a Catholic university. The Spiritans, a Catholic missionary community of priests, brothers, and laity, founded Duquesne University in 1878. The Spiritan spirituality, or Charism, and principals of Catholic social teaching shape the focus of service-learning at Duquesne. Specifically, because the Spiritan mission is carried out by engaging in the concrete struggles of society, faculty find administrative support for creating service-learning opportunities that focus on working for social justice and human dignity; core principles of the Spiritan Charism (Koren, 1990).

EVOLUTION OF SERVICE-LEARNING WITHIN THE OCCUPATIONAL THERAPY CURRICULUM

The occupational therapy curriculum at Duquesne University is a five-year entry-level master's degree program. Service-learning is a key teaching pedagogy and has been integrated at several levels throughout the curriculum. Much like the early days of the service-learning pedagogy in education (Dewey, 1938; Kolb, 1984) and in the education of health professionals (Tai-Seale, 2000), early efforts involved integrating "experiential learning" and "service opportunities" into several courses in the curriculum. At that point, our efforts emphasized service and volunteerism for the specific purpose of providing students with professional development opportunities. For example, students were generally encouraged to find a community agency without occupational therapy services where they could practice their group leadership and clinical reasoning skills. Over the years, students found many community agencies that were open to their enthusiasm and efforts to implement group sessions for their consumers. Community agencies were willing to host the students for a short-term, six-week project and were grateful for student involvement with the population they served. As faculty studied and embraced service-learning pedagogy, a more thoughtful and intentional application of service-learning principles was developed. In the following sections, we present a developmental application of service-learning experiences. The reader should be mindful that this current sequence is a result of years of refinement and ongoing adaptations to maximize effectiveness of service-learning.

The current approach, embedded in the design of service-learning opportunities, combines conscious-raising, guided reflection, and thoughtful planning for advocacy and action on issues of occupational and social justice. Occupational justice is "the promotion of social and economic change to increase individual, community, and political awareness, resources, and equitable opportunities for diverse occupational opportunities which enable people to meet their potential and experience well-being" (Wilcock, 1998, p. 257). Guided reflections are prompts that call students to pause and consider the relationship between the learning goals and service goals and between theory taught in the classroom and actual practice. For example, during the first of three semesters of service-learning (Clinical Reasoning I), when students are getting to know the population they are serving, the guided reflection questions simply ask the students to describe what they observed, what it means, and what the next steps should be. These guided reflection questions might be as simple as "What?", "So what?", and "Now what?" This set of questions challenges students to use their observational skills and process what they have observed. At the beginning of the next semester, the questions become a bit more specific and challenge students to link the service experience with topics or theory in discussed in class. For example, students might be asked: "Describe how you are using your narrative reasoning skills to better understand the issues, concerns, and needs your client is facing?" or "How will you apply what you have learned about the client to next week's session?" Finally, at the end of the second semester of this service-learning project, students respond to a question such as this: "Through this experience, you have demonstrated that you are an engaged citizen. You advocated on behalf of the population you served in service-learning. In particular, you advocated on behalf Frank, Mark, Ryan, Rob, Dave, Mike, Susan, Kathy, Tamara, and others. You gave voice to their needs. Describe the significance of this advocacy experience to you. Describe the significance of completing your service-learning project in this way." Table 5-1 provides a summary of how guided reflections are incorporated throughout the curriculum.

Specific assignments, journaling, lectures, roundtable discussions with community partners, and regular and sustained engagement with consumers in the community are consistent components of our approach. The sequence of courses in the curriculum and the developmental continuum of major service-learning objectives connected to each course are presented in Table 5-2.

Learning objectives integrated into service-learning in early semesters focus on applying foundational knowledge and building a basic practice skill set. Courses in subsequent semesters provide

Table 5-1 Guided Reflections Throughout the Curriculum.

Year and OT Courses	Service-Learning Objectives/Activities	Sample Reflection Questions
4th year, Fall: Clinical Reasoning I	• Spend time observing and getting to know the population and site. • Conduct informal needs assessment.	• "What?" • "So what?" • "Now what?" • Students describe what they have observed, what it means, and next steps.
4th year, Spring: First half of Clinical Reasoning II	• Provide 10-week group interventions. • Include weekly feedback survey from participants.	• Describe how you are using your narrative reasoning skills to better understand the issues, concerns, and needs your client is facing. • How do you apply what you have learned about the client to next week's session?
4th year, Spring: Last reflection Clinical Reasoning II	• Participate in an advocacy trip to Washington D.C. on behalf of population served. • Meet with legislators. • Give voice to population's concerns and needs.	Through this experience, you have demonstrated you are an engaged citizen. You advocated on behalf of the population you served in service-learning. You advocated on behalf of Frank, Mark, Ryan, Tamara, and others. You gave voice to their needs. • Describe the significance of this advocacy experience to you. • Describe the significance of completing your service-learning project with an advocacy trip.
5th year, Summer: Community and World Health	• Conduct more extensive needs assessment. • Develop a program. • Write a grant to support program. • Present program and grant to community agency.	• Describe how this summer's experience in the community (whether or not you plan to work in a community setting) has influenced your understanding of your vocation, your calling as an occupational therapist. • How has this summer experience helped you to understand your gifts and talents?

Table 5-2 Service-Learning Objectives Across the Curriculum.

	Being With and Finding Voice	
Semester	Course	Service-Learning Objectives Integrated into Course
3rd year, Fall	Fundamentals of Practice	• Understand occupational profile. • Develop interviewing skills. • Reflective practitioner skills. • Support listening project research.
4th year, Summer	Human Groups and Occupation	• Explore personal behavior, feelings, and reactions to clinical and nonclinical interpersonal situations. • Design and implement therapeutic group sessions. • Demonstrate effective group leadership. • Document accurate observations.

	Doing With and Giving Voice	
Semester	Course	Service-Learning Objectives Integrated into Course
4th year, Fall	Clinical Reasoning and Fieldwork IA	• Understand clinical reasoning skills. • Apply OT process skills. • Apply basic clinical reasoning skills. • Demonstrate professional written/verbal skills.
4th year, Spring	Clinical Reasoning and Fieldwork IB	• Demonstrate knowledge and application of clinical reasoning concepts and skills. • Demonstrate relationship among person, environment, and occupational performance. • Analyze data and evidence gathered as emerging practice scholar. • Design consumer education materials.

	Advocacy and Joining Voice	
Semester	Course	Service-Learning Objectives Integrated into Course
5th year, Summer	Occupational Therapy Administration	• Produce a comprehensive occupational therapy program proposal for the community agency based upon the needs expressed by the staff and the clients served.

(continued)

Table 5-2 (*Continued*)

Semester	Course	Service-Learning Objectives Integrated into Course
		• Develop an understanding of an occupational therapist's responsibilities in a community site. • Analyze how an occupational therapist fits within the organizational structure of the community agency. • Develop a job description for an occupational therapist as well as a performance assessment based on the job description.
5th year, Summer	Community and World Healthcare Issues	• Construct an in-depth understanding of a given community by producing a program plan that considers a variety of factors (e.g., economic, cultural, political) influencing healthcare delivery. • Obtain and analyze vital demographic and health status data for specific populations and/or health issues. • Design community-based programs that include occupational therapy roles that move beyond direct treatment paradigms (e.g., consultation, case management, advocacy, and education).
5th year, Summer	Evidence-Based Practice	• Demonstrate ability to communicate research evidence to a variety of stakeholders, including colleagues, consumers, and community partners. • Generate descriptive assessment and intervention effectiveness questions relative to assigned community-based programs. • Locate, evaluate, and synthesize research evidence to substantiate proposals for person-centered, evidence-based occupational therapy programming.

opportunities for students to apply a knowledge base that, through coursework, grows in depth and breadth. Service-learning experiences offer opportunities for real-world practice of a broad repertoire of skills that support clinical practice, the development of community partnerships, and practice scholarship (Lorenzo, Duncan,

Buchanan, & Alsop, 2006; Muñoz, Provident, & Witchger Hansen, 2005; Witchger Hansen, Muñoz, Crist, Gupta, Ideishi, Primeau, et al. 2007). The culminating service-learning event in our curriculum challenges students to integrate knowledge and skills they are developing in the final three courses they complete before embarking on their Level II fieldwork. This capstone learning project demands a high level of collaboration and the capacity to engage independently in a self-directed process of inquiry that supports the students' continued transformation into lifelong learners. The guided reflective exercises are designed to assist students to not only develop their own voice as a health professional, but also to cultivate their ability to investigate, analyze, and act to address healthcare disparities experienced by populations that are marginalized in our society.

BEING WITH AND FINDING VOICE

A consistent component at each level of service-learning is the use of guided reflection. Reflective exercises are designed to assist students to not only develop their own voice as a health professional, but also to cultivate their ability to investigate, analyze, and address healthcare disparities experienced by populations that are marginalized in our society. This approach to learning is informed by the authors' reviews of student reflections. We have noted some consistent patterns about how students describe their lived experience of these service-learning opportunities. Students use reflective journaling to process their experiences. They document shifts in their own understanding of the challenges of living in poverty, the struggle to remain in recovery, or the constant energy one needs to avoid and resist the negative aspects of their physical and social environments. Their reflections on the lives of others frequently generate an introspective evaluation of their own lives. Their journal entries often indicate not only a broader knowledge of the community context, but also document the development of their own sense of self and voice (Belenky, Clinchy, Goldberger, & Tarule, 1997). Our observations of the impact of service-learning programs on these students' self-concept, sociopolitical engagement, and attitudes toward marginalized groups are similar to those documented in the service-learning literature (Morgan & Streb, 2001; Gadbury-Amyot, Simmer-Beck, McCunniff, Williams, 2006).

As faculty, we have found that at this point in their development as health professionals, most students view health care through the lens of a middle-class health service delivery model: Healthcare services are delivered in a clean doctor's office or well-provisioned hospital. For most students at this level, issues such as access, quality of care, health disparities, the influences of poverty on health, or stigma and marginalization are largely unknown. The earliest service-learning opportunities in our curriculum are designed to help students listen to the voices of marginalized populations as they describe their lived experiences with these issues. Reflective journaling exercises provide structure to assist students in finding their own voice to express what they are learning about the healthcare needs of marginalized populations and to thoughtfully consider occupational therapy's role in addressing these needs (Bringle & Hatcher, 1997; Daudelin, 1996).

FUNDAMENTALS OF PRACTICE VOICES

Service-learning opportunities begin in the Fundamentals of Practice course and are designed to address a relevant community-identified need. For example, this past year, 2008, the course instructor uncovered a community need during an environmental scan and community exploration of our university neighborhood. The Quakers were seeking volunteers to interview and record the military stories of returning war veterans for their community-sponsored Military Listening Project, located at a local shelter for homeless war veterans located several blocks from campus. This experience was designed to provide the listening project with interviewers, while addressing a course objective—to enhance the students' listening and interviewing skills. While documenting the experiences of returning veterans, the students learned about the health and occupational performance challenges these veterans face (Bringle & Hatcher, 1996; Israel & Ilvento, 1995).

The Military Listening Project uses a process of ethnographic interviewing to elicit stories from veterans, their families, and community service workers about the challenges of postdeployment reintegration (American Friends Service Committee, 2007). After a formal orientation of the local Military Listening Project, provided by a community partner, students work in pairs and meet and interview returning war veterans at a convenient, nonthreatening environment; a local shelter for war veterans who are experiencing homelessness. Initial interviews use a semi-structured interview guide to collect data for the Military Listening Project's ongoing research. These questions focus on the challenges that veterans' experience coming back from war, including how their return has impacted their home life, family relations, and employment situation. Health problems and experiences with military health service delivery are also key components of these interviews (American Friends Service Committee, 2007). Additional questions, designed by the students and instructor, help students generate an occupational profile of the veteran. Using the OPHI-II (Kielhofner et al., 2004) as a guideline, the students document the veteran's occupational profile. Thus, the service-learning objective in this course, to address a community-identified need while enhancing interviewing skills, is designed to help students develop interview skills while simultaneously addressing a community-identified need—documenting the experiences of returning veterans and learning about the health and occupational performance challenges these veterans face (Bringle & Hatcher, 1996; Israel & Ilvento, 1995).

Again, guided reflection questions are used to help students process and mark the development of their own skills, knowledge, and attitudes. Effective reflection activities link service with learning objectives, are guided, occur regularly, allow feedback and assessment, and clarify values (Hatcher, Bringle, & Muthiah, 2004).

Reflection is guided by prompts such as "Describe what was significant about this experience," and "How did this experience affect your development as an occupational therapist?" One student responded to such questions with the following journal entry:

> The idea of interviewing a veteran first made me quite anxious.
> I was unsure what I would say, if I'd become emotional, and
> if the veteran would open up during the process. After conducting the interview and meeting the Marine veteran, who
> was a resident of Shepherd's Heart, I realized what a wonderful experience it truly was, forever changing the way I view
> different types of people, particularly the homeless. . . I am
> very appreciative of being able to have met M and learn more
> about the life he lives. His positive attitude despite being
> homeless impacted me greatly, proving that it takes more than
> material goods to be happy; something that we all know but
> sometimes forget. It also allowed me to practice interviewing
> someone, just as I would a client in the future.

The focus on selecting community sites that will move students
out of the university context and that create opportunities for engaging diverse populations is an intentional pedagogical strategy
(Lohman & Aitken, 2002; Campinha-Bacote, 2003; Muñoz, 2007).
Such cross-cultural encounters offer the opportunity for students
to develop the skills, knowledge, and attitudes that support culturally responsive caring (Campinha-Bacote, 2003; Muñoz, 2007). The
following student's reflection addresses how these encounters not
only created an opportunity to listen to and give voice to someone
they might not have ever made the opportunity to listen to if not
for the service-learning experience, but also how these encounters
provided the opportunity to develop practice skills:

> I think that this interview hugely helped me not only in my
> actual interview skills, which I will undoubtedly use in my career, but by giving me the opportunity to meet someone new
> and very different from myself. When I am working as an occupational therapist, most of my clients will be extremely different than me and each other. I will need to be able to see each
> of them as individuals, who have thoughts, feelings, and needs
> different from my own. Only by understanding this, will I be
> able to treat clients to the best of my ability, with the best

possible results. Being able to talk to M enabled me to see a homeless person and veteran for whom they are, not only a statistic, which is a priceless experience.

HUMANS, GROUPS, AND OCCUPATIONS VOICE

The next opportunity for students to find their own voice as healthcare professionals comes in the summer of the fourth year in their Humans, Groups, and Occupations course. This course examines theories and practice of effective interpersonal communication and group processes for therapeutic, supervisory, and professional functions. In collaboration with a community liaison, the students complete a needs assessment and then design groups that address a health or occupation need for populations served at a selected community agency. For example, for the past two years students have designed and implemented groups at the Woodlands, an independent-living center for children and adults with disability and chronic illnesses (Woodlands Foundation, 2008). Students are challenged to design group protocols and individual sessions consistent with a specific occupational therapy practice model, such as the model of human occupation or the occupational performance model. This course is structured so students are on-site at the Woodlands at least twice weekly for four consecutive weeks. Each student leads or coleads up to eight group sessions addressing areas such as prevocation, social skills training, life skills and IADL training, and relaxation and coping. Students are challenged to reflect on their own development as a group leader and also learn to document their clinical observations using a SOAP note format.

DOING WITH AND SHARING VOICE THROUGH CLINICAL REASONING

Students' service-learning experiences in the Fundamentals and Humans, Groups, and Occupations courses create opportunities designed to assist their development of a broader view of health care and their own identity as a health professional. Over the next two semesters, we build upon this foundation with service-learning events in the Clinical Reasoning I and II courses.

These courses are based on learning and service objectives, specifically (1) demonstrate knowledge of clinical reasoning concepts through understanding the occupational performance needs of a particular vulnerable population and (2) articulate the relationship among person, environment, and occupational performance by developing a service-learning proposal that addresses a community-identified need. Service-learning activities begin with the students spending three hours a week for six weeks in a community agency getting to know the vulnerable population they are serving and the population's occupational performance needs. Using the data collected from these weekly experiences and through informal (conversation and observation) and formal (COPM, Kawa River, OPHI-II) encounters, students discuss their findings with the community agency staff and develop a program proposal that addresses these identified needs. In a roundtable format at the community agency in the last week of the fall semester, students present their program proposal and timeline to the community agency staff and instructor and together discuss its feasibility and implementation plan for the Spring semester. If the community agency determines the project is unrealistic, the students will join another service-learning group. If the community agency agrees to host the project, students meet before the semester break to plan for implementation of the program in January.

In January, during Clinical Reasoning II, students carry out the 8- to 10-week project. The project includes conducting appropriate pre- and post-assessments with each program participant, carrying out a weekly group or individual intervention, and collecting evidence and outcomes from these efforts. In tandem with these service projects, students are addressing community-identified needs, learning and practicing more advanced clinical reasoning skills, as well as learning about and addressing issues of social and occupational justices through an advocacy project. Learning and service goals for this phase of the project include the following:

- Demonstrate the use of clinical reasoning skills, including procedural, interactive, and conditional reasoning in identifying and evaluating patient/client occupational performance issues while addressing community-identified needs of a vulnerable population during service-learning.

- Demonstrate the capacity to work in partnership with a community agency to creatively address the occupational performance needs of the population they are serving.
- Utilize self-reflection to develop insight into how one contributes to or detracts from the therapeutic partnership with service-learning population.
- Articulate understanding of the concepts of social justice, occupational alienation, deprivation, and imbalance as observed in the context of the community setting.

For the past several years, students have participated in an integrated, client-centered, occupation-focused service-learning experience. This experience requires a sustained community partnership that extends for approximately 10 months. The instructor in these courses specifically chooses community agencies that serve vulnerable populations. For example, students are placed at community correction centers serving ex-offenders (Renewal Inc., 2006); drop-in mental health centers (Fifth Avenue Commons, 2005); shelters for homeless men and women (Bethlehem Haven, 2007; Light of Life Rescue Mission, 2007); and community centers for disabled veterans dealing with issues of poverty, substance abuse, and mental illness (Shepherd's Heart, 2008). As stated earlier, community partnerships are developed over time by faculty conducting ongoing environmental scans, neighborhood walking tours, and discussions with university colleagues also involved in community-based service-learning projects.

Collaboration on service-learning objectives within these Clinical Reasoning courses requires the course instructor to touch base with the designated community agency service-learning supervisor by e-mail or phone at least weekly and students fulfilling their required three-hour weekly activity at their assigned site. This weekly communication with the instructor helps to establish structure and supports that facilitate successful community service-learning experiences (Giles & Eyler, 1994; Honnet & Poulen, 1989; Shumer, 1997).

Key service-learning assignments include the completion of a community agency profile based on a thorough needs assessment of the community agency and the development of an intervention program that meets a defined need of the population using approaches supported by research evidence.

Clinical Reasoning I and II are structured to ensure the students' weekly participation in activities at their community site. For example, students are required to document the hours they spend in the community agency and the specific weekly activities that they provide for the program participants. Service-learning assignments in the first semester emphasize the development of a project proposal. This proposal takes shape through an iterative process of collaboration with community partners and culminates in a roundtable discussion at the end of this first semester where students and their community partners strategize project outcomes and timelines for the next semester. The collaborative process inherent in completing a needs assessment and planning the project ensures that the students' projects meet community-defined needs. The students' consistent and sustained participation at the community agency combined with the instructor's regular communication with the community agency liaison ensures a successful partnership whereby expectations and outcomes are clearly negotiated (Giles & Eyler, 1994; Honnet & Poulen, 1989; Shumer, 1997).

In the second course of this sequence (Clinical Reasoning II), students and their service-learning supervisors revisit the implementation plan. Once the plan is approved, students carry out their project, typically some type of life skills, health and wellness, or job preparation group sessions. In the course of completing their projects, students conduct assessments, develop individualized and group goals, plan group intervention sessions, document their weekly observations, and conduct reassessments. They also collect outcomes evidence from the programs they implement. This focus on outcomes measurement plants the seeds of practice scholarship and generates potential research questions or programming possibilities that can be pursued in future service-learning experiences. Throughout the semester, as students study advanced issues in clinical reasoning and topics such as spirituality, occupational justice, social justice, resilience and hope, ethics, and dealing with difficult patients, they reflect on their service-learning experiences in light of their understanding of these concepts.

Over the years, we have learned to carefully craft the activities we use to bring closure to this and every set of service-learning experiences. We expect students to present the outcomes of their project and to process their experience with their community partners. These presentations are always held at the agency and are open to agency staff and consumers alike. Successful community partnership requires an intentional respect for the culture of each community partner and the populations they serve (Suarez-Balcazar, Muñoz, & Fisher, 2006). Efforts to build this level of mutuality and reciprocity opens the door for future service-learning collaborations.

The next step in our developmental progression of service-learning events requires students to write program proposals for new occupational therapy services that are grounded in the research evidence, and to submit this proposal in the structure of a basic grant application. Details of this capstone experience are provided in the following section.

ADVOCACY AND JOINING VOICES

The capstone service-learning event in our curriculum occurs as students reach their graduate year of education. Our efforts in this year focus on helping students build knowledge, skills, and confidence in their role as healthcare professionals. Three key features distinguish the heightened expectations for service-learning outcomes in this semester. The first is that students must strengthen their own voice by assuming roles that address population-based healthcare needs. The second is that they must hone their skills of consultation and take pivotal roles in facilitating the generation of a shared vision of program development with their community partners. The third feature is that a single service-learning experience is integrated across three courses. Key learning events in each course are designed to produce scholarly products that, when combined, result in the generation of one comprehensive service-learning project. Course activities in an Occupational Therapy Administration course, a Community and World Health course, and an Evidence-Based Practice course are integrated to structure this service-learning experience. The courses described here are the only courses delivered in the summer semester of the student's fifth year in our entry-level master's program.

All three courses are designed as graduate seminars and each meets three times a week for two and a half hours. In two of the courses, the schedule is structured so that students routinely meet at their assigned community agency rather than in the classroom to facilitate relationship-building and to contextualize the learning. The rationale to integrate these three courses arose from several sources. First and foremost was a genuine desire to provide students a capstone experience that builds upon their earlier service-learning experiences. It is our goal to develop professionals who are prepared to forge their own paths in a community health context that is dynamic and challenging. The integration of these three courses and active collaboration with our partners at nonprofit community agencies allows us to embed the major learning assignments in these courses in community-based service-learning experiences. In our experience, we have learned that creating a three-semester thread of service-learning at the same agency offers students, agency staff, and service-learning consumers time to develop meaningful, trusting relationships. We train our students to serve as ambassadors from our occupational therapy department and the profession. As such, they play a key role in opening doors for future collaborations and in advocating for the profession. Finally, we are motivated to create service-learning opportunities that serve as transitional events between the classroom environment and clinical practice. This service-learning experience directly precedes Level II fieldwork. We designed this service-learning experience to prepare students for the significant role transition from classroom student to fieldwork student.

Occupational Therapy Administration

The Occupational Therapy Administration course aims to provide students with an introduction to the basic principles of designing and administrating occupational therapy programs. The course covers topics related to planning, budgeting, quality management, staffing, and program development. Upon completion of this course, students are expected to differentiate between managers and leaders; identify various forms of organizational structure; describe the human resource process with respect to recruitment, interviewing, and candidate selection; and create and critique performance evaluations.

The major learning assignments in this course include: (1) development of a proposed occupational therapy program for an assigned community agency, (2) creation of a professional resume, and (3) identification and discussion of contemporary administrative issues. The students learn to market themselves as unique professionals based upon the work they are doing with the agency. They look at various styles of resumes and perform mock interviews while receiving peer and professional feedback. Students also survey current newspapers and online sites to discuss contemporary examples of managerial situations that are occurring in the complex world of health care.

The program development assignment, prior to the collaboration of the authors, was a group project where the students created a *hypothetical* occupational therapy program containing the following major sections: general purpose, mission statement, SWOT analysis, program description, needs assessment, budget, organizational structure, implementation plan, position description, performance standards, marketing plan, and program evaluation. This program development assignment assisted students in developing competencies relative to administration, but it did not offer the students the opportunity to gain the experience and feedback needed to test the viability of their program ideas in a real-world context. Since the initial collaboration of the authors and subsequent refinement of the assignments into service-learning objectives, current students are assigned the task of developing a feasible program for their assigned community agency based upon a completed needs assessment generated in the Clinical Reasoning courses the semester prior. The students then work together in groups of three to four with the objective of determining a viable program to meet the stated needs of the agency and its consumers.

This major service-learning assignment constitutes 40% of the students' final grade and needs to include several separate, yet intercoordinated, sections of a comprehensive program proposal. Upon completion of their work, each group turns in a professional package portraying their proposed occupational therapy program. Each program proposal must include the components shown in Table 5-3. The students are responsible for developing all necessary forms and language that is consistent with the agency for all sections of the proposal. By requiring consistency in look and language of what is already being used by the community site, the students begin to join the voice of the agency and several outcomes result. First, the students need to continually communicate with the leaders in the agency, which give the students the responsibility of preparing for the meetings and establishing timely and consistent communication with the staff. Additionally, by mandating that the forms, language, and marketing look of the products are consistent with the agency's, the likelihood that the program will be accepted and implemented is greater, because the transition would be minimal from concept to implementation.

The students produce this comprehensive program proposal with the input of the executive directors and staff of the agencies. The final copy of the program proposal is given to the agency to determine if it would like to pursue the program. The results of this educational strategy have produced over 50 program proposals since the inception of the educational collaboration. These programs have been proposed in 25 different community agencies, ranging from the local YMCA to shelters serving the homeless and senior citizen centers offering adult day services.

Community and World Health

The Community and World Health course focuses on building competencies for community-based practice and covers topics such as community assessment; models of community practice; grant writing and funding for community practice; community-based programming; indirect service delivery models, such as consultation, case management, and education; and cross-cultural and international perspectives on healthcare delivery. Class sessions

Table 5-3 Administration Program Proposal Subsections.

Program Component	Content
General purpose	The unique purpose of the program is outlined to describe the general areas to be covered, based upon identified needs of the agency and clients served.
Mission statement	A concise statement designed for the proposed program which includes the philosophical rationale for the program. This statement should be powerful and inclusive of the purpose of the program. The mission statement of the program should be congruent with the mission of the agency.
SWOT analysis	The Strengths, Weaknesses, Opportunities, and Threats are identified and outlined for the program. Internal issues that support or deter the agency from using the proposed program as well as external competitors and community assessment data are identified.
Program description	Hours of operation, setting, population to be served, as well as the level of personnel delivering the content are outlined. General information about the program content is emphasized and thoroughly explained.
Needs assessment	The key needs are identified, determined through assessment of clients, personnel, and or staff at the facility.
Budget	Realistic financial estimates for three years are outlined and a projected budget covering both operational and capital needs and how monetary figures were determined are explained.
Organizational structure	Key persons and positions are identified within the agency and presented within the organizational chart. The new occupational therapist for the proposed program is fit into the existing organizational structure.
Implementation plan	A timeline demonstrating the key needs for implementation of the program taking into consideration realistic time frames as well as inclusion of all needs for start up of the program.

(*continued*)

Table 5-3 (*Continued*)

Program Component	Content
Position description	A comprehensive occupational therapy position description is written, which fits into the overall program as stated in the design and program description. This position description includes all major job responsibilities and includes ADA (Americans with Disability Act) appropriate language.
Performance standards	Standards to evaluate the occupational therapist's performance are developed according to the position description. Performance criteria that are objective and able to be measured are created. A performance appraisal form consistent with the agency's performance reporting system is developed.
Marketing plan	A plan that is eye-catching and descriptive of the program, including a logo or slogan that is consistent with marketing the image of their program is developed and used on all sections of the program proposal. The plan to market the program must be based upon the financial situation of the agency and the proposed budget.
Program evaluation	An evaluation plan that assesses the outcomes of the program, taking into consideration the mission and philosophy, and that includes methods to carry out the program evaluation is designed. It also identifies who will be responsible in carrying out the evaluation.

typically cover content relative to community health care and incorporate active learning exercises in the classroom, computer labs, or in the community. One class session per week is dedicated to providing time for students to meet with the executive director or staff at their assigned community agency. During these meetings, students complete structured experiential exercises in data collection, program development, and grant writing.

Course learning activities are designed to assist students in identifying, synthesizing, and reporting data that serve as indicators of community health. Students examine demographic and epidemiologic data, track educational trends and economic development within the community, and analyze the availability of health, social, and recreation services. These tasks challenge students to communicate with a variety of public and governmental agencies to gather and interpret relevant data. Learning activities are designed to help students understand how to analyze the vital demographic and health status data they have collected about a specific community. At a broader level, students are challenged to compare and contrast the healthcare delivery systems of major industrialized and nonindustrialized nations and to examine the role of occupational therapy within these systems. They review major national healthcare policy issues, including disease prevention and health promotion policies, and consider future healthcare trends and the possible impact of these trends on occupational therapy and other health professions.

The major learning assignments in Community and World Health include: (1) a community assets map through a walking and "windshield tour"; (2) a community agency profile, including a needs assessment of the agency and surrounding community; and (3) a basic grant application focused on funding the program the students have designed in their Occupational Therapy Administration course. In addition, students are required to complete guided reflections to document the experience of developing competencies for community-based practice.

As a first step, students are encouraged to become familiar with the local context of the agency by exploring the local community and creating a "community assets map." Students often take a walking tour of the community and a "windshield" (driving) tour of the local area to gain a broad understanding of the community context and health resources. Students use ethnographic observation skills to observe the activities and daily routines of the community agency they have been assigned, its programs, and the consumers who access these programs. They design interviews and use these to gather data from the agency's executive director and staff and consumers. Students use a detailed outline to conduct a thorough needs assessment (see Table 5-4).

Table 5-4 Community Agency Profile Content.

Profile Component	Content
Contact information	Facility, address, executive director, phone, e-mail, Web site
Organizational profile	History, mission and goals of the organization, organizational structure, funding sources, communities served, significant recent successes, significant future challenges, agency's relationship to community, key community partners
Programs and services profile	Consumer demographics, referral procedures, program staff, major programs and services, most/least successful programs, marketing methods, results of agency's needs assessment
Program evaluation and research context profile	Program evaluation methods, research context, ongoing studies, overall research climate
Community partners profile	Potential community partners (that could add depth or breadth to any new program proposal)
University partners profile	Potential Duquesne University partners (that could add depth or breadth to any new program proposal), faculty input, health science student input
Opportunities for community–university partnership	Duquesne University Occupational Therapy Department (two ways the OT Department might consider partnering with this agency and how learning objectives in classroom can be extended into this community setting)
Community profile: Ethnographic	Data collection, observations in the community, summary/analysis of participant observations in the agency, summary/analysis of surveys/interview(s) with executive director and program director, summary/analysis of surveys/interview(s)/focus groups with staff, summary/analysis of surveys/interview(s)/focus groups with consumers

(*continued*)

Table 5-4 (*Continued*)

Profile Component	Content
Relevant epidemiologic data for the community	Epidemiological data, data sources (U.S. or PA census, agency reports, Department of Health and Human Services, Department of Public Health, etc.)
Program/service needs	Three potential program/service needs identified in needs assessment
Relevant evidence/best practices	Three annotated sources, evidence of best practices. For each study include: (1) APA citation; (2) population description; and (3) key findings
Relationship to Healthy People 2010 initiatives	Specific connection to Healthy People 2010 objectives
Potential funding sources	Foundation sources, state/federal sources

They complete similar tasks at other agencies in the community that address similar populations or that offer supporting services to similar consumer groups so that they can gain a holistic understanding of the population's needs and the community resources available to address those needs. In weekly dialogue with the agency and course instructors, students uncover the occupational performance needs of a specific population served by the community agency and develop a program proposal, budget, and implementation timeline. Simultaneously, students research the literature to find evidence to support their program proposal.

Each student group prepares a basic grant application that incorporates elements of their program proposal and uses the supporting evidence they have uncovered in the needs assessment and the literature. Completing the grant application challenges the students to synthesize data from multiple sources, including the program proposal they have developed, the research evidence they have located to support their program interventions, and details of the program's implementation, including space, personnel, and budgetary needs. Their challenge is to produce a well-organized, concise grant proposal that includes an engaging cover letter, executive summary, clear program description, and an efficient budget and outcomes measurement plan. Finally, students identify at least three foundations and/or "request for proposals" that might serve as potential funders of their proposed program. At the end of the semester, the products from key learning assignments across these courses are delivered to the community agency during a presentation and roundtable discussion at the agency. Each agency is a left both hard and electronic copies of all materials.

Evidence-Based Practice

The Evidence-Based Practice course is designed to provide opportunities for students to apply and extend knowledge acquired in qualitative and quantitative research methods courses and to strengthen their ability to analyze and evaluate evidence that supports the practice of occupational therapy. Principles relative to evidence-based practice are covered in short lectures, and the bulk of the learning is structured in guided discussion of research and critical appraisal of evidence and outcome measurement in small group and journal club formats. Student in this course learn by doing; class sessions often begin or end in a computer lab where students use sites such as OTSeeker, SumSearch, the Cochrane Databases, and AOTA's Evidence-Based Practice Briefs, to find evidence that may help them answer questions defined by the instructor or in collaboration with community partners.

Course learning activities are designed to assist students in applying specific performance skills for locating, organizing, evaluating, and using research evidence. Every intervention course in the curriculum emphasizes the development of these skills, and this course demands higher level performances for analyzing and evaluating research evidence. Additionally, students are challenged to generate new ways of designing and producing reports of the evidence they have uncovered. Specifically, they are challenged to communicate the results of their analyses in written executive summary and program description sections of a common grant application and in written and verbal presentations to community agency consumers, staff, and executive directors.

As stated, this course is designed as a graduate seminar, and learning objectives are met using a variety of teaching/learning methods, including guided discussions, journal club presentations, peer-to-peer critiques, and hands-on exercises in computer labs and in the community. A journal club is built into the structure of this graduate seminar to create an opportunity for students to synthesize, discuss, and critique research literature and to share and defend their analyses with their peers. As in many such courses, student learning is supported with assignments that expect effective search patterns and critical appraisal of the evidence as well as challenges that test the students' abilities to effectively communicate their findings.

Service-learning adds a critical "real-world" dimension to the learning events designed in this course. For example, when students hone their ability to generate descriptive, assessment, and intervention effectiveness questions (Tickle-Degnen, 2008), this process is grounded in the concerns and program needs of their assigned community-based service-learning site. For example, a student group assigned to a community corrections site serving exoffenders defined the following questions:

1. What are the critical components of effective vocational integration programs? (descriptive question)
2. What are effective tools for measuring community reintegration as an outcome? (assessment question)
3. Is supportive employment an effective approach for helping exoffenders find and keep competitive employment? (intervention question)

At the end of the semester, a presentation to the community agency directors, staff, and consumers creates an opportunity for students to demonstrate the skills necessary for verbally communicating their synthesis of outcomes using language that is meaningful and useful to the various stakeholders (Eyler, Giles, Stenson, & Gray, 2001).

COMMUNITY PARTNERSHIP

The seeds for developing partnerships with community agencies were planted more than a decade ago when the Occupational Therapy Department was founded. The Duquesne University curriculum is designed to integrate service-learning projects and experiential class assignments that place students into community agencies serving various populations, such as at-risk youth; physically and mentally challenged men, women, and children; homeless and/or incarcerated populations; and the frail elderly.

One method we use to measure outcomes for our service-learning assignments is to solicit written feedback from agency or program directors at our community partnership sites to continue to perfect the application of this pedagogy. The feedback we have received is overwhelmingly positive. Most agencies report that the program proposals meet defined needs of the populations they serve. Almost all agree that they would implement the program and hire an occupational therapist if they could secure funding for the position. Some agency directors pointed out that a relative weakness in the grant proposals was the accuracy of the budget projections. Feedback from executive directors, agency staff, and consumers on both the process and products of the service-learning experience has helped us continually refine our service-learning collaborations.

Additionally, we seek student feedback at the conclusion of the semester through anonymous postcourse evaluations so that the process can be continually analyzed for its effectiveness and usefulness to the students. Again, feedback was mostly positive. Students reported that they felt the projects helped them develop a deeper understanding of the context of community practice and had increased their capacity and confidence to create their own community-based position. Students also remark that they are more aware of the foundations that fund health care and alternative ways to support occupational therapy services and that the assignments demystified the grant-writing process. However, although students report an increased investment in their projects because it had a "real-life" application, they continued to question whether the agency would consider moving forward on their proposal. The pessimism expressed by some students offers an opportunity for a teachable moment about the fiscal realities of community-based occupational therapy practice. Exploration of these concerns allows for frank discussions of how best to advocate for occupational therapy services. Further, solution-focused discussions help highlight the critical need to integrate reliable and accurate program and individual outcome measures into the design of their program proposals.

Brainstorming strategies for generating evidence that occupational therapy is effective provides instructors with the opportunity to nurture these students' identities as practice scholars.

LESSONS LEARNED FROM SERVICE-LEARNING

Like all occupational therapy faculty, our faculty routinely evaluate our curriculum and teaching methods. Given the prominent role service-learning plays in meeting learning outcomes in our curriculum, we specifically examine the service-learning experiences we have created. We synthesize feedback and routinely question how learning events can be adapted. We also examine the community–university partnerships we have developed, and, although we stay open to new opportunities, we have learned that depth in a few partnerships leads to better outcomes than having multiple community contacts that we cannot hope to effectively sustain. As educators, we draw on many sources as we strive to employ best educational practices in service-learning (Honnet & Paulson, 1989; Eyler & Giles, 1999; Mintz & Hesser, 1996; McGowan, 2002; Lohman & Aitken, 2002; Marstellar & Kowaleski, 2005).

We make a conscious effort to develop our craft as educators and explore works that may provide us with innovative frameworks for thinking about effective community-based service-learning (Lorenzo et al., 2006). We are also mindful of integrating learning-centered approaches that lead us to consistently question what types of learning will be significant for our students (Fink, 2003). Our intentional selection of community sites that serve the most marginalized members of our society lead us to draw on many works that elucidate strategies for walking the talk of occupational therapy's social vision (Kronenberg et al., 2005; Watson & Swartz, 2004).

Our work is founded in a collaborative process that intentionally applies service-learning pedagogy and concretely connects learning and service objectives in multiple courses throughout our curriculum. Our challenge has been to create learning events that are designed and delivered in such a way that discovery and skill development in one class supports synthesis and application in the next. The development of this strategy continues today as an iterative and reflective process. Critical reflection on our educational strategies is informed by feedback and outcome data from the students and the community agencies with whom we have partnered.

Through the development of this collaborative over the years, we have learned, and continue to learn, from our successes. Frequently, some of the most useful lessons have come when projects have not worked out as we might have hoped. The lessons we have learned over the years, mirror what others have reported (Bringle & Hatcher, 1996; Bringle & Hatcher, 1999; Connors, Cora-Bramble, Hart, Sebastian, & Seifer 1996; Witchger Hansen et al., 2007). The following are some reflections on what we have learned.

Communication

The key to the success of service-learning assignments rests in effective communication between the students and the community agency throughout each step of the process. From the initial meeting with the community agency staff and "service-learning supervisor" to discuss learning and service goals, to interviewing staff and consumers for the needs assessment and analysis, to program development and writing the grant, students are required to communicate personally and electronically every week. During these weekly meetings at the community agency, students process their findings with their service-learning supervisor, seek clarification, and determine next steps collaboratively. Oftentimes, students find they have misinterpreted a conversation with a staff member and, very quickly, assume their project should morph into a direction that is not appropriate based on this small but important misinterpretation. Weekly meetings with their service-learning supervisor keep both the agency and the students "on track." We have also learned that a single point of contact between the community and university partners facilitates clear and direct communication and creates the type of reciprocal relationships that supports effective problem solving.

Creating a "Just Right" Challenge

Over the past 15 years of implementing service-learning into various courses within our occupational therapy curriculum, we have learned important lessons on how to create the "just right" challenge for the students and how to develop and maintain effective community–university partnerships to support service-learning. We learned these lessons through listening to the voices of our students in their weekly reflections, course evaluations, and teacher effectiveness reviews. In addition, we learned lessons from ongoing communication with our community partners, community partner evaluations of projects, and faculty peer reflection and assessment of our experiences throughout the semester and at the end of each semester, when we meet together as a team to review our experiences.

We have learned that each semester we have a new cohort of students and that it is useful to take into consideration each student group's unique strengths, experiences, and interests, as well as the strengths and needs of our community partners, before assigning students to a partner and a particular site. Some semesters we allow students to choose their own partner and the site within a prearranged group of community agencies; sometimes we, as faculty, based on our understanding of the students' strengths and characteristics of the agency infrastructure, assign students to a particular partner. At the beginning of each semester, instructors sit down together to discuss which community partners we will choose for the coming semester, any adjustments to learning activities based on our recent experiences, and how we will encourage ongoing effective communication between the students and their host sites.

Choosing Community Partners in Advance

Educators cannot underestimate the key role that preplanning plays in successful service-learning experiences. Such planning ensures that students can "hit the ground running" at the beginning of the semester. We have found that considering the strength of the community agency's infrastructure (particularly staff availability to supervise), staff openness to student partners, appropriateness of community-identified service needs to student learning needs, and access to staff and consumers, as well as a willingness to spend time with our students each week are basic criteria to follow in choosing community partners.

Aware of the core characteristics of effective community–university partnerships identified by the field (Community-Campus Partnerships for Health, 1998; Torres, 2000; Honnet & Poulsen, 1989), we have found similarities with our experiences. Although each of these lists of characteristics was created to reflect unique aspects of their contexts, "there is a high level of convergence in their recommendations that proves a vision of ideal partnerships" (Sandy & Holland, 2006, p. 34). In our experience, we have learned distinct lessons regarding community–university partnerships for service-learning, many of which mirror the work of Sandy and Holland (2006).

Sustaining Relationships with Our Community Partners

In the end, what makes any partnership work are the relationships we build with our community partners. To this end, we have found that personal contact with our community partners from the beginning, each sharing our expectations, learning and service objectives, and hope for outcomes ensures that we are all working toward common goals and expectations. Through this process of ongoing personal and electronic communication, we develop a sense of mutual trust and organizational commitment, the key to our mutual success. In addition, we share our syllabi and course objectives with our community partners to ensure that they have an understanding of why this partnership and project is an important component of student learning. Through ongoing discussion, we ensure that we both have mutually agreed upon goals. We also share the rewards. In presentations to professional audiences, faculty recognize the contributions of our partners, and in some cases our partners have presented with us in these venues. In a similar vein, when we can support our partners by describing our collaborations in meetings with their board of directors or funding agencies, we make sure to prioritize these events.

We have also learned that many community agencies wish to be more engaged with the course content through technology. We ask all of our partners if they are interested in accessing our course readings, syllabus, and schedule through Blackboard. Many of our community partners want to be connected in this way. When they request this connection, we establish them as a "guest" of our Blackboard site and welcome them to contact us by e-mail or through the online discussion board. It is through collaborations with our students, community agency staff, and the clients they serve, that we strive to keep the voices heard and keep service-learning an active dynamic component of our occupational therapy curriculum.

Through collaboration with our students, community agency staff, and the clients they serve, we begin by listening to the voices in our community to understand their needs. Then, we create programs that address their community-identified needs, sharing their voice and doing with them. And finally, through our collaborative efforts, we join our voices with theirs, advocating for their needs, and raising our voices in a creative service-learning collaboration to address the needs of marginalized populations as an active and dynamic component of our occupational therapy curriculum.

References

American Friends Service Committee. (2007). The human cost of war: Listening to voices of Iraq veterans and their families from recruitment to post deployment. Retrieved February 1, 2008, from http://www.afsc.org/pittsburgh/documents/MLPreport2.pdf.

American Occupational Therapy Association. (1993). Core values and attitudes of occupational therapy practice. *American Journal of Occupational Therapy, 47,* 1085–1086.

American Occupational Therapy Association. (1995). The philosophical base of occupational therapy. *American Journal of Occupational Therapy, 49,* 1026.

American Occupational Therapy Association. (2002). Occupational therapy practice framework: Domain and process. *American Journal of Occupational Therapy, 56,* 609–639.

American Occupational Therapy Association. (2005). Occupational therapy code of ethics (2005). *American Journal of Occupational Therapy, 59*(6), 639–641.

Belenky, M. F., Clinchy, B. M., Goldberger, N. R., & Tarule, J. M. (1997). *Women's way of knowing: The development of self, voice & mind.* New York: Basic Books.

Bethlehem Haven. (2007). Bethlehem Haven: Changing lives for good. Retrieved February 7, 2008, from http://www.bethlehemhaven.org/.

Bickford, D., & Reynolds, N. (2002). Activism and service learning: Reframing volunteerism as acts of dissent. *Pedagogy, 2*(2), 229–252.

Boyer, E. (1994, March 4). Creating the new American college. *Chronicle of Higher Education, 9,* A48.

Bringle, R. G., & Hatcher, J. A. (1996). Implementing service-learning in higher education. *Journal of Higher Education, 67*(2), 221–239.

Bringle, R., & Hatcher, J. (1997). Reflection: Bridging the gap between service and learning. *College Teaching, 45*(4), 153–158.

Bringle, R. G., & Hatcher, J. A. (1999). Reflection in service-learning: Making meaning of experience. *Educational Horizons, 77*(4), 179–185.

Campinha-Bacote, J. (2003). *The process of cultural competence in the delivery of healthcare services,* 4th ed. Cincinnati, Ohio: Transcultural C.A.R.E. Associates.

Community-Campus Partnerships for Health. (1998). Principles of good community-campus partnerships. Seattle: Author. Retrieved December 8, 2004, from http://depts.washington.edu/ccph/principles.html#principles.

Connors, K., Cora-Bramble, K., Hart, R., Sebastian, J., & Seifer, S. (1996). Interdisciplinary collaboration in service-learning: Lessons from the health professions. *Michigan Journal of Community Service-Learning, 3,* 113–127.

Cuban, S., & Anderson, A. (2007) Where's the justice in service-learning? Institutionalizing service-learning from a social justice perspective. *Equity & Excellence in Education, 40,* 144–155.

Daudelin, M. W. (1996). Learning from experience through reflection. *Organizational Dynamics, 24*(3), 36–48.

Dewey, J. (1938). *Experience and education.* New York: Collier.

Duquesne University, Department of Occupational Therapy. (n.d.). Mission. Retrieved January 15, 2008, from, http://www.healthsciences.duq.edu/ot/hb03history.html.

Eyler, J. S., Giles, D. E., Stenson, C., & Gray, C. (2001). *At a glance: What we know about the effects of service-learning on college students, faculty, institutions, and communities.* Nashville, TN: The Vanderbilt University.

Eyler, J. S., & Giles, D. E. (1999). Where's the learning in service-learning? San Francisco: Jossey-Bass.

Fifth Avenue Commons. (2005). Fifth avenue commons: A collaborative community. Retrieved February 7, 2008, from http://www.alleghenycounty.us/uploadedFiles/DHS/About_DHS/Publications/Resource_Guides/FifthAvenueCommonsDirectory.pdf.

Fink, L. D. (2003). *Creating significant service learning experiences.* San Francisco: Jossey-Bass.

Gadbury-Amyot, C. C., Simmer-Beck, M., McCunniff, M., & Williams, K. B. (2006). Using a multifaceted approach including community-based service-learning to enrich formal ethics instruction in a dental school. *Dental Education, 70*(6), 652–661.

Giles, D. E. Jr., & Eyler, J. (1994). Theoretical roots of service learning in John Dewey: Toward a theory of service learning. *Michigan Journal of Community Service Learning,* Fall, 77–85.

Hatcher, J. A., Bringle, R. G., & Muthiah, R. (2004). Designing effective reflection: What matters to service-learning? *Michigan Journal of Community Service-Learning, 11*(1), 38–46.

Honnet, E. P., & Poulsen, S. (1989). *Principles of good practice in combining service and learning: Wingspread special report.* Racine, WI: Johnson Foundation.

Israel, G., & Ilvento, T. (1995). Everybody wins: Involving youth in community needs assessment. *Journal of Extension, 33,* 2.

Kielhofner, G. (2004). *Conceptual foundations of occupational therapy.* Philadelphia: F. A. Davis.

Kielhofner, G., Mallison, T., Crawford, C., Nowak, M., Rigby, M., Henry, A., et al. (2004). *Occupational Performance History Interview II (OPHI-II) Version 2.1.* Available online at http://www.moho.uic.edu/assess/ophi%202.1.html.

Kolb, D. A. (1984). *Experiential learning: Experience as a source of learning and development.* Englewood Cliffs, NJ: Prentice-Hall.

Koren, J. (1990). *Essays on the Spiritan charism and on Spiritan history.* Bethel Park, PA: Spiritus Press.

Kronenberg, F., Algado, S. S., & Pollard, N. (Eds.). (2005). *Occupational therapy without borders.* Philadelphia: Elsevier Churchill Livingstone.

Light of Life Rescue Mission. (2007). A community where broken people find hope. Retrieved February 7, 2008, from http://www.lightoflife.org/.

Lohman, H., & Aitken, M. J. (2002). Occupational therapy students' attitudes toward service learning. *Physical & Occupational Therapy in Geriatrics, 20*(3/4), 155–164.

Lorenzo, T., Duncan, M., Buchanan, H., & Alsop, A. (2006). *Practice and service learning in occupational therapy: Enhancing potential in context.* Hoboken, NJ: John Wiley & Sons.

Marstellar, B., & Kowaleski, B. (2005, August). ASA academic workshop: Approaches to service learning. Paper presented at the meeting of the American Sociological Association, Philadelphia, PA.

McGowan, T. G. (2002). Toward an assessment-based approach to service-learning course design. In R. Devine, J. A. Favazza, & F. M. McLain (Eds.), From cloister to commons: Concepts and models for service-learning in religious studies (pp. 83–91). Washington, DC: American Association for Higher Education.

Mintz, S., & Hesser, G. (1996). Principles of good practice in service learning. In B. Jacoby (Ed.), *Service learning in higher education: Concepts and practices* (pp. 26–52). San Francisco: Jossey-Bass.

Morgan, W., & Streb, M. (2001) Building citizenship: How student voice in service-learning develops civic values. *Social Sciences Quarterly, 82*(1), 154–169.

Muñoz, J. P. (2007). Culturally responsive caring in occupational therapy. *Occupational Therapy International, 14*(4), 256–280.

Muñoz, J. P., Provident, I., & Witchger Hansen, A. (2005). Educating for community-based practice: A collaborative strategy. *Occupational Therapy in Health Care, 18*(1/2), 151–169.

Renewal Incorporated. (2006, October). Your guide to resident services, Version 5.0. Retrieved February 7, 2008, from http://www.cor.state.pa.us/ccc/lib/ccc/Renewal.pdf.

Rimmerman, C. (1997). *The new citizenship: Unconventional politics, activism and service.* Boulder, CO: Westview.

Sandy, M., & Holland, B. (2006). Different worlds and common ground: Community partner perspectives on campus-community partnerships. *Michigan Journal of Community Service Learning, 13*(1), 30–43.

Shepherd's Heart. (2008). Shepherd's Heart Veterans Home. Retrieved February 7, 2008, from http://shepheart.com/luke/.

Shumer, R. (1997). Learning from qualitative research. In A. Waterman (Ed.), *Service-learning: Applications from the research.* Mahwah, NJ: Lawrence Earlbaum Associates, Inc.

Suarez-Balcazar, Y., Muñoz, J. P., & Fisher, G. (2006). Building culturally competent community–university partnerships for occupational therapy scholarship and practice. In G. Kielhofner (Ed.), *Research in occupational therapy: Methods of inquiry for enhancing practice* (pp. 632–642). Philadelphia: F. A. Davis.

Tai-Seale, T. (2000). Service learning: Historical roots, present forms, and educational potential for training health educators. *Journal of Health Education, 31*(5), 256–261.

Tickle-Degnen, L. (2008). Communicating evidence to clients, managers and funders. In M. Law & J. MacDermid (Eds.), *Evidence-based rehabilitation: A guide to practice,* 2nd ed. (pp. 263–296). Thorofare, NJ: Slack.

Townsend, E. (1993). Muriel Driver lecture: Occupational therapy's social vision. *Canadian Journal of Occupational Therapy, 60,* 174–184.

Townsend, T., & Whiteford, G. (2005). A participatory occupational justice framework. In F. Kronenberg, S. S. Algado, & N. Pollard (Eds.), *Occupational therapy without borders,* (pp. 110–126). London: Elsevier Inc.

Torres, J. (Ed.). (2000). *Benchmarks for campus/community partnerships.* Providence, RI: Campus Compact.

Wade, R. (2001). *And justice for all: Community service-learning for social justice.* Issue paper for the Education Commission of the States. Retrieved May 7, 2008, from http://ecs.org/clearinghouse/29/13/2913.htm.

Watson, R., & Swartz, L. (2004). *Transformation through occupation.* London: Whurr Publishers.

Westheimer, J., & Kahne, J. (2004). What kind of citizen? The politics of education for democracy. *American Educational Research Journal, 41*(2), 237–269.

Western Pennsylvania Grant Makers. (2008). Common grant application format. Retrieved February 8, 2008, from http://www.cmu.edu/giving/files/common-grant.pdf.

Wilcock, A. (1998). *An occupational perspective of health.* Thorofare, NJ: Slack.

Witchger Hansen, A. M., Muñoz, J. P., Crist, P., Gupta, J., Ideishi, R., Primeau, L. A., et al. (2007). Service learning: Meaningful, community-centered professional skill development for occupational therapy students. *Occupational Therapy in Health Care, 1–2,* 25–49.

Woodlands Foundation. (2008). Retrieved February 5, 2008, from http://www.woodlandsfoundation.org/.

Yerxa, E. (1983). Audacious values: The energy source for occupational therapy practice. In G. Keilhofner (Ed.), *Health through occupation: Theory and practice in occupational therapy.* Philadelphia: F. A. Davis.

Chapter 6

Service-Learning, Health Promotion, and Occupational Therapy: A Good Fit

Callie Watson, OTD, OTR/L
Kristin Haas, OTD, OTR/L

Health promotion, as defined by the World Health Organization, is the process of enabling people to increase control over and to improve their health (WHO, 2008). Minkler (1997) states that in the United States *health promotion* is much more narrowly defined as "the science and art of helping people change their lifestyle to move toward a state of optimal health" (p. 7). The profession of occupational therapy asserts that health and wellness are related outcomes to the key outcome of occupational therapy intervention: enhancing engagement in occupation.

The *Occupational Therapy Practice Framework: Domain and Process* (OTPF) (AOTA, 2002) defines *health,* based on the WHO definition, as "a complete state of physical, mental, and social well-being and not just the absence of disease or infirmity" (WHO, 1947, p. 29). Health and wellness occupational outcomes are similarly aligned with outcomes for participation, prevention, and quality of life identified by the World Health Organization (WHO, 2001). The OTPF identifies prevention of illness, disease, injury, or disability is an important outcome of occupational intervention at individual, group, and societal levels to facilitate healthy behaviors and lifestyles (AOTA, 2002). Quality of life is related to an individual's sense of satisfaction, health status and functioning, and life participation (AOTA, 2002).

An awareness of one's own health values and beliefs as well as knowledge and skills in the concepts of health and health promotion are necessary competencies for occupational therapy students entering the healthcare field. The Accreditation Council For Occupational Therapy Education (ACOTE) requires occupational therapy educators to provide students with learning experiences that enhance their knowledge not only of health and health promotion but also their understanding of social, cultural, economic, and political contexts of health and disability in order to facilitate a multicultural perspective of health for individuals across the lifespan (ACOTE, 2008). Additionally, students need to understand, implement, and evaluate occupational therapy service models that incorporate individuals, groups, and the community (ACOTE, 2008). Furthermore, the Pew Health Professions Commission (1998) outlined recommendations for healthcare education in stating, "Health professional programs should require a significant amount of work in community settings, students should assist in the design and development of community programming" (p. 5). Based on these mandates, the occupational therapy faculty at College of Saint Mary (CSM) chose to incorporate service-learning and community-engagement pedagogies and experiences as part of an occupational therapy course on health promotion.

Through the health promotion course at CSM, students are provided an opportunity to design, implement, and evaluate occupation-based health promotion interventions and assess the outcomes of these interventions with various community agencies. This is an excellent fit for occupational therapy students, faculty, community agencies, and the institutional organization of CSM. Students are able to practice specific skills sets used by occupational therapists while contributing to the health and wellness of participants from various community agencies.

This chapter focuses on how CSM faculty in the occupational therapy department planned and implemented a service-learning health promotion program. This course and program originated in the community and involved a partnership between four community organizations and the Department of Occupational Therapy as a means of providing needed services with the community and providing occupational therapy students with experiential educational and community training activities.

SERVICE-LEARNING FOR STUDENTS, FACULTY, COLLEGES, AND COMMUNITIES

In a comprehensive review of the literature, Eyler, Giles, Stenson, and Gray (2001), found that participation in service-learning courses positively impacted student outcomes in terms of personal development, social benefits, advances in learning, career development, and improved relationships with their college or institution. Research conducted by RMC Research (2006) found that students who participated in service-learning reported greater increases in pro-social behaviors, such as altruism, caring, respect, and the ability to choose between right and wrong, than their peers in the comparison group. Numerous studies have shown that participation in service-learning courses at institutions of higher education benefits students, faculty, the institution, and the community (Eyler et al., 2001).

Research also suggests that faculty, as well as colleges and universities, are increasingly integrating service-learning into courses and committing themselves to service-learning (National Association of State Universities and Land Grant Colleges, 1995; Stanton, 1994; Ward, 2000). The literature also suggests favorable outcomes for faculty incorporating service-learning. For example, faculty who use service-learning report satisfaction with the quality of student learning (Balazadeh, 1996; Berson & Younkin, 1998; Cohen & Kinsey, 1994; Calleson, Parker, & Morgan, 1996; Ward, 2000). Moreover, Driscoll, Holland, Gelmon, and Kerrigan (1996) reported that faculty state a commitment to research after integrating service-learning into curriculum.

Benefits from service-learning extend beyond institutions of higher learning into the community. Numerous studies have found that communities are satisfied with student participation (Clarke, 2000; Ward & Vernon, 1999; National Association of State Universities and Land Grant Colleges, 1995). Service-learning was also found to be useful in communities, as outlined by a report from Western Washington University in 1994. This research helps to validate service-learning's place in the learning environment.

Thoughtful planning by faculty and the community is essential for successful learning and partnerships that meet course and community goals and are sustainable over time. The following section will discuss strategies for planning service-learning experiences.

GETTING STARTED, MEETING THE MISSION, AND PREPLANNING

Studies have suggested that the quality of course content matters to students (Billig, 2006). Characteristics such as a strong link between service-learning activities and content standards, direct contact with those being served, cognitively challenging reflection activities, student choice in planning and implementation of activities, and implementing service-learning for the entire semester are vitally important to student outcomes (Ash, Clayton, & Atkinson, 2005; Astin & Sax, 1998; Astin, Vogelgesang, Ikeda, & Yee, 2000; Eyler & Giles, 1999; Ikeda, 1999).

At CMS, the instructors prepared an action plan using the template in Table 6-1 prior to their Spring 2008 Health Promotion course (Table 6-1). Faculty had learned from past service-learning courses that an action plan is essential when working with outside agencies and collaborating with students and faculty. Communication is

Table 6-1 Action Plan Template.

Action Steps	Resources	Who Is Responsible?	Timeline
Grant writing	Grant writer on campus	Callie and grant writer	Date
Contact community agencies			
Meet with agencies			
Choose appropriate agencies			
Develop course syllabus			

vitally important in making sure the course and the community relationships are on target. The course was co-taught; therefore, coordination was needed between faculty and the community agencies involved.

The action plan included finding agencies that fit or matched well with the CSM mission (see Appendix 6-B), finding community agencies in need of health promotion, and finding and securing grant funds to reach more community needs. In the fall of 2007, the faculty applied for a grant from the Omaha Urban AHEC (Area Health Education Center) Community Grant.

After the grant was written, the faculty met with the service-learning coordinator at the college to see about matching up with community partners already developed within the college. Following this meeting and after investigating other community agencies, the faculty selected and evaluated the possibilities. Faculty met with numerous agencies and shared philosophies, ideas, and missions. In doing service-learning across the curriculum, faculty have learned the importance in preplanning and taking time to ensure that each facility is matched well with the college and the course learning objectives. Table 6-2 shows the selection process checklist created by faculty.

Table 6-2 Selection Process Checklist.

Selecting a Partner That Fits with Your Institution, Program, and Course Needs

Relationship can be ongoing	Yes	No
Facility has commitment for students	Yes	No
Reciprocal learning can occur	Yes	No
Mission of facility supports course objectives	Yes	No
Share commitment to a common vision	Yes	No
Appear to be collaborative and open	Yes	No
Does the facility understand concept of service-learning?	Yes	No
Can the work at the facility be the just right challenge?	Yes	No

In keeping with our mission (see Appendix 6-B), CSM's occupational therapy program engages students in service to the community that improves their skills and knowledge and prepares them to be leaders in their field. We believe that we can combine this goal with our compassionate service to others in the community to assist students in becoming the best occupational therapy practitioners they can be and prepare them for an outstanding career in the field.

It is important to always link service-learning assignments (or any other teaching modality) to the mission of your college. This helps in getting support for the program on a higher level. After meeting and spending some time at each agency, the faculty agreed upon the final four agencies in which the students would be doing health promotion training, life skills education, and health career promotion. The agencies chosen included the Women's Care Center of the Heartland (WCCH), Mercy Housing, the Morton Magnet School, and the Ollie Webb Center.

It was after this that the faculty learned that they had been awarded the Omaha Urban AHEC (Area Health Education Center) Community Grant, totaling $5,500 to be split among the community agencies. AHEC prides itself on educating and inspiring underrepresented students' interest in careers in the health professions, as well as encouraging healthcare professionals, in providing equitable and quality services to disadvantaged and underserved populations. Faculty felt the agency's mission was in line with the mission of CSM and the occupational therapy department.

Next, faculty developed the course syllabus (see Appendix 6-A) and developed rubrics and reflection strategies for both students and community agencies. Establishment of grading criteria and expectations, as well as well-thought-out outcomes, in the preplanning stages helps to guide everyone involved.

Implementation of a modified logic model to assist with program planning and evaluation is also a part of the preplanning stages. Faculty at CSM feel strongly that a (modified) logic model is essential in developing appropriate and measurable indicators during the planning phase and is key to sound evaluation of what you are trying to accomplish in service-learning. Logic models are tools that can aide in describing the effectiveness of a service-learning program and have been used for more than 20 years by program evaluators to describe the effectiveness of their programs (McCawley, 2008). Logic models "illustrate a sequence of cause and effect relationships—a systems approach to communicate the path towards a desired result" (Millar, Simeone, Carnevale, 2001, p. 73).

Faculty developed the modified logic model in Table 6-3 to view outcomes related to this experience. Table 6-4 shows the modified logic model for the Women's Care Center health promotion objectives. Note that these examples are not full logic models.

The logic model is helpful in the preplanning phases to convey the fundamental purpose of the service-learning, to demonstrate why the service is important and, most important, to depict the actions and causes expected from the experience. Creating the logic model prior to visiting with agencies ensures that you have a solid foundation of what you expect from your students and the community partners. Developing appropriate and measurable indicators during the preplanning phase can be pivotal to a sound evaluation of service-learning.

Table 6-3 Modified Logic Model I.

Objective	Evaluation Method	Evaluators
Students will survey patients and community agencies.	Assess appropriateness and effectiveness of assessment tool.	Dr. Haas and Dr. Watson
Students will analyze needs and prepare sessions.	Ensure that analysis matches stated needs.	Dr. Haas and Dr. Watson
Students' curriculum will reflect indicated needs.	Ensure that curriculum addresses stated needs.	Dr. Haas and Dr. Watson
Students' curriculum will factor in socioeconomic and sociocultural needs.	Ensure that curriculum addresses specific population needs.	Dr. Haas and Dr. Watson
Students will describe learning in weekly reflection journals.	Quality and depth of reflection.	Dr. Haas and Dr. Watson
Students' curriculum will offer a variety of life skills sessions.	Ensure that curriculum provides variety and provides training on appropriate life skills.	Dr. Haas and Dr. Watson
Students will take pretests and post-tests.	Gather information regarding students' self-concept and self-evaluation of skills and compare between tests.	Dr. Haas and Dr. Watson Students
Students will write and publish about their experience	Acceptance of articles for publication.	Editorial board of various journals
Students will articulate in their weekly journals the need for serving all populations.	Quality and depth of reflection.	Dr. Haas and Dr. Watson Students
Students will develop a plan to serve.	Realistic and thoughtful plan.	Dr. Haas and Dr. Watson

Table 6-4 Modified Logic Model II.

Goals	Activities	Objectives (Outcomes)	Indicators	Who Evaluated	Data Sources	Data Analysis
WCCH residents will be more likely to eat healthier.	Students and residents will collaboratively participate in cooking and nutrition life skill groups 12 times in 2 months.	Residents will develop long-term plan and desire for healthier eating. Residents will acquire knowledge about nutrition and healthier eating habits.	All residents will complete life skills (cooking) groups. Residents will change previous eating habits to selecting and cooking healthier.	Residents	Interviews and observations	Self-reports and comparisons
WCCH residents will increase self-concept and develop self-advocacy skills.	WCC residents will participate in self-esteem/advocacy life skills group three times in two months.	Residents will be able to identify three or more statements regarding self and be able to articulate one need for self appropriately.	Residents will complete self-concept and advocacy life skill groups. Residents will identify three positive aspects of self and articulate one need for self appropriately.	Residents	Interviews and observations	Self-reports and comparisons

(*continued*)

Table 6-4 (*Continued*)

Goals	Activities	Objectives (Outcomes)	Indicators	Who Evaluated	Data Sources	Data Analysis
CSM students will learn group therapy techniques based on frames of references in OT.	Students will plan and run life skill groups 12 times in 2 months.	Students will acquire knowledge on group leadership skills and group dynamics.	Students will successfully complete all life skills groups.	Students	Observation, rubrics, interviews, and journals	Self-report documentation
CSM students will demonstrate knowledge and appreciation of role of sociocultural, socioeconomic, diversity factors and lifestyle choices in contemporary society.	Students will plan and run life skill groups to homeless pregnant women.	Students will acquire knowledge and appreciation of different backgrounds.	Students will articulate appreciation of role of sociocultural, socioeconomic, diversity factors and lifestyle choices in contemporary society.	Students	Observation, interviews, and journals	Comparison, reflections, documentation
CSM students will learn the value to serve.	Students will plan and run life skill groups to homeless pregnant women.	Students will articulate need for serving all populations and develop plan to serve in future.	Students will serve in future.	Students	Interviews and surveys	Self-reports

HEALTH PROMOTION COURSE OBJECTIVES AND CONTENT

The health promotion service-learning program had the following goals and objectives for the students involved:

1. Students will employ logical thinking, critical analysis, problem solving, and creativity in health promotion and patient/community education.
   - Students will survey patients and community agencies to assess health promotion needs.
   - Students will analyze needs and prepare health promotion and career exploration sessions based on needs.
   - Students' curriculum will reflect the indicated needs.
2. Students will demonstrate knowledge of and appreciation for the role of sociocultural issues, socioeconomic factors, diversity factors, and lifestyle choices in patients.
   - Students' curriculum will factor in the socioeconomic and sociocultural needs of their patients.
   - Students will describe the learning that takes place in their weekly reflection journals.
3. Students will promote the importance of life skills balance to the achievement of health and wellness.
   - Students' curriculum will offer a variety of life skills sessions that can attribute to patients' health and wellness.
4. Students will increase self-concept and develop professional skills.
   - Students will take a pre-test prior to working with the clients of the four agencies and a post-test at the end of the course.
   - Students will write and publish about their experience.
5. Students will learn the value of service to others.
   - Students will articulate in their weekly journals the need for serving all populations.
   - Students will develop a plan to serve in the future.

During the first six weeks of the semester, students studied health promotion intensively. (The syllabus and specific course topics are provided in Appendix 6-A.) Other topics presented during this period were service-learning, the concept of community, peer assessment, group dynamics, and the performance of a mini needs analysis. One class period was set aside to enable the students to visit each community agency for an orientation session, including tours of the facility and a discussion of the agency's mission and philosophy statements. Students were then required to rank the sites in the order in which they would like to work with them and to justify their selections. Based on this information, the faculty split students into groups for each facility. After their justifications, the students were asked to reflect on their thoughts about service-learning, health promotion, and their work in the community.

We strive to have the students do authentic and meaningful work in the community, so why not have their writing in the classroom be authentic and meaningful as well? In this service-learning course, students are required to publish an article concerning occupational therapy, health promotion, a topic they are passionate about, and/or service-learning. Students usually begin the writing process with hesitation, unaware that they have the skills needed to be published. Students are encouraged to seek out their own publication interests, and faculty help guide and facilitate the writing of papers, establishment of objectives, and publication efforts. By doing this, students will come to appreciate the importance of publishing and understand the need to informing the public about occupational therapy and health promotion.

MINI NEEDS ANALYSIS

Ensuring that the authentic needs of the community agencies are being met is essential in developing and sustaining long-lasting relationships. The students were instructed on how to complete a mini needs analysis during the first six weeks of the course. The students and faculty assessed the health needs and developed a corresponding curriculum for residents of the Women's Care Center of the Heartland (WCCH) and Mercy Housing as well as for the students of Morton Magnet Middle School and clients of the Ollie Webb Center. Students completed a Strengths, Weaknesses, Opportunities, and Threats (SWOT) analysis on each facility. They surveyed all stakeholders to ensure that the community agency's needs were met. Students conducted assessments and interviews to acquire information about the health needs of the clients and then analyzed the results and developed life skills and health promotion sessions addressing the stated and assessed needs (see Table 6-5). Students then created a health promotion and health career curriculum centered on the guiding principles of health promotion: advocacy for health, enabling people to achieve their fullest health potential, strengthening communities, and developing personal social skills to achieve better health.

Table 6-5 Sample Needs Analysis Rubric.

A. Overview of the Facility: Provide a detailed description of the clients the facility it serves, location, space availability etc.	5 points
B. How long has the facility been in existence? How is it funded? Where is it located and why? What is its mission? How is it meeting its mission? What programs are currently offered? Who is offering them?	5 points
C. Program Development: Provide a brief statement as to the need of a program at this facility. What if any research is there to justify such a program?	10 points
D. SWOT Analysis: Complete a SWOT analysis ON THIS PROGRAM/PROJECT: 1. What are the strengths of the facility (internal)? 2. What are its weaknesses (internal)? 3. What are opportunities for the facility (external)? 4. What are potential threats for the facility (external)?	10 points
E. Program Goals: What are your goals for your program? Include specific time frames. Are your time frames realistic? How will you know if you met your goals? Who will run this program?	5 points
F. Strategies: What are the specific strategies used to meet each of the goals?	5 points
G. Program Evaluation: How will you monitor if your program is effective? How often will you evaluate your program? Who will complete the data collection and how will they store the data?	5 points
H. References (APA format)	5 points

Note that students also took into account the socioeconomic and sociocultural factors and lifestyle choices of the clients they served. These important aspects were taken into consideration when developing curriculums at each site in order to ensure that the educational materials and training sessions are sensitive to those issues and are culturally competent. It is imperative for occupational therapy students to have the ability to work well with patients from a wide variety of backgrounds with diverse health issues and needs and varying socioeconomic statuses and experiences. However, without experiences in the field working with clients, many do not attain these skill sets and learning experiences before they graduate. As you have read, service-learning is an excellent modality to assist students in achieving accreditation standards. By actually doing and experiencing occupational therapy skills, processes, and methods, students develop their critical-thinking skills as well as discover clinical reasoning skills. After the seventh week of the semester, the students spent their time at the community agencies until the end of the semester providing health promotion and health career promotion.

It is imperative to provide the community agency with resources that will extend longer than just the experience during the semester. Therefore, through the needs analysis and program planning, students are responsible for coming up with long-lasting resources for the agency. The resources the faculty and students provide are excellent ongoing outcomes for the program.

COMMUNITY SITES UTILIZED IN THE HEALTH PROMOTION COURSE

The following is a brief overview of the community agencies that were utilized in conjunction with this course and grant.

Women's Care Center of the Heartland (WCCH)

The WCCH provides support in a residential setting for homeless women during and after pregnancy. While at the center, the women attend parenting classes and meet with the Family Life Director to create a plan with goals for themselves. All of the women's pregnancy and birth needs are met. The women range from 19 to 23 years of age. Women come from diverse socioeconomic and sociocultural backgrounds.

Students who selected WCCH provided life skills training sessions that included information on nutrition, budgeting, time management, education on a safe and healthy pregnancy and post pregnancy, job readiness and interviewing skills, and career/college exploration. According to WCCH staff, the women have expressed concern about leaving their supportive environment and making it on their own. As a way to meet this need, students compiled a resource manual for residents who leave the facility. It includes information on housing; free health, dental and vision clinics; free activities in the area, as well as childcare and self-care resources. This will be a resource the facility can distribute for years after the students leave.

Mercy Housing (Focusing on Mason Apartments)

Mercy Housing, Inc. was established to provide better and more comprehensive housing programs than previously accessible and is now one of the largest housing organizations in the United States, providing housing development, property operations, and management services. Founded in Omaha, Nebraska, in 1981, the idea quickly took hold elsewhere, expanding to 42 states and the District of Columbia and now serving more than 75,000 people (Sisters of Mercy, 2008). Mercy Housing's mission is to create stable, vibrant and healthy communities by developing, financing and operating affordable, program-enriched housing for families, seniors, and people with special needs who lack the economic resources to access quality, safe housing opportunities. The average family size at Mason Apartments is six; the median yearly income is $12,000; ethnicity is 80% Sudanese, 10% African American, and 10% Caucasian.

CSM students provided crucial health promotion and life skill topics to the residents, both mothers and children at the Mason apartments. A curriculum resource guide focusing on good nutrition and healthy families was left with Mercy Housing staff to implement after students have left the agency.

Morton Magnet Middle School: Center for Community Research and Design

Morton Magnet Middle School's mission is to develop a commitment to learning and the personal success of each student in the school. The school seeks to provide a caring atmosphere to ease the transition from elementary school to middle school while developing critical-thinking skills, fostering acceptance of responsibility, and improving academic performance through the recognition of individual learning styles. The magnet theme at Morton is community, research, and design. In conjunction with academics, Morton Magnet Middle School guides its students toward developing a sense of self-worth, good character, active citizenship, good health, and an awareness of lifetime work and leisure options. The school encourages an awareness and understanding of other cultural heritages and respect for the diversity found in school and society.

At Morton Magnet Middle School, CSM students created a health promotion and career exploration curriculum and provided skills set training sessions throughout the semester. Students also created marketing materials for administrators to help showcase their magnet. The elective health promotion course the students developed was entitled: College of Saint Mary (CSM) presents Morton I.D.O.L.S, which stands for "individual development of life skills." CSM occupational therapy students and faculty assisted Morton students in selecting health promotion activities and field trips to participate in during the last 10 weeks of their semester. In addition, the CSM students and Morton students planned a service-learning field trip to do together.

Ollie Webb Center

Ollie Webb's mission is to enrich the lives of individuals with developmental disabilities and their families through support, programs, and advocacy. Ollie Webb offers a broad range of programs to accomplish its mission. Additionally, it is a resource for current information on disabilities and disability law. CSM students provided health promotion and life skills training to adults 18 and older in the continuing education classes at the Ollie Webb Center. CSM students facilitated evening classes for adult or adolescent populations who are either in school or at work during the day. Finally CSM students developed a mentoring program at CSM for any student to work with a client of Ollie Webb on a one-on-one basis. This was put in place to ensure a longer-lasting relationship with the Ollie Webb Center.

CSM students worked with individuals with developmental disabilities (DD). Many individuals with developmental disabilities tend to become obese as they age, specifically people those with Down syndrome and Prader-Willi syndrome (Lisa Dougherty, personal communication, 2008). The participants not only learned health promotion skills, but also the valuable skill of socialization. Many times individuals who have developmental disabilities only interact with their families or other individuals with developmental disabilities. Any opportunity for them to interact with members of the community is an opportunity to work on their social skills (e.g., introducing themselves, appropriate conversation topics, eye contact, etc.). Another benefit is that they may increase their self-esteem and self-confidence. If they are aware that these students are interested in and excited to work with them, they may feel like an accepted part of a group or community The CSM students, in turn, benefited from being with the diverse group of individuals.

Students worked with a diverse mix of people at Ollie Webb Center, including those with Down syndrome, autism, and a variety of learning disabilities. This allows the students to put their textbook knowledge to work in the "real world." The CSM students were able to have a positive experience and increase their self-esteem and self-confidence in knowing that they were helping others.

OUTCOMES AND REFLECTIONS

Assessment is important in evaluating the effectiveness of service-learning. Through assessment, faculty members are able to examine the contributions made by service-learning and document the work of the students as evidence to various stakeholders of the college (and community). The modified logic model helps in determining the effectiveness of the experience. We have found that the learning that takes place far extends the objectives set forth in the classroom and the modified logic model.

It is also important to look at outcomes that do extend beyond the modified logic model. Outcomes for this particular course included the opportunity to present the service-learning course to various local and national conferences. Faculty members at CSM were selected to present within their college, to colleagues, at a Mercy Conference, and at a national magnet conference. CSM faculty and one teacher and one administrator from the middle school were accepted to present at the Magnet Schools of America 26th Annual National Conference. This presentation highlighted the partnership of Morton Magnet Middle School and the College of Saint Mary, including the innovative curriculum design and theme integration.

Student Reflections

Research suggests that structured or guided opportunities for reflection enable the student to gain a deeper understanding and construct their own meaning from the experience (Moon, 1999). In this service-learning course, faculty used Eyler and Giles (1999) effective strategies for fostering reflection as a template for guided reflections throughout the learning experience. Eyler and Giles (1999) describe reflection as being continuous, connected, challenging, and contextualized. Therefore, the students were asked to reflect after the first day of class. The following are some of the students' pre-reflections:

- "I personally think the service-learning project sounds like a great and rewarding opportunity. I think it will benefit both us as students and those we help in the community. I am excited to get out there and start this project."
- "Upon hearing about the service-learning assignment for our Health Promotion Class, I became very excited! I think it will be an awesome experience all around! It has the opportunity

of offering new friendships, new cultures/lifestyles, and most of all a hands-on learning experience."

- "I feel excited and scared at the same time. Excited to go out into the community and have a chance to really make a difference in that community. At the same time it's a little scary because I keep thinking to myself, "can I really do this?" Can I really go out and help create a program for a community that has the potential to be long lasting and have a wonderful impact on the community I get to service?"
- "Right now I am feeling both excited and nervous about service in the community. I want to learn new skills, develop my own therapeutic-use-of-self (so that I can be effective and confident while still being respectful and contextual). I am also excited about working with new classmates and helping others identifies truly meaningful and perhaps life-changing, objectives/goals."

Students were also asked to reflect before attending the sites on what their goals and objectives for the service-learning project might be. The following are examples of student goals:

- "Confidence"
- "I would like to learn how to problem solve in different situations while learning about the community. I want to learn more about different ways of promoting health and have resources to utilize the information."
- "How to interact with people from different backgrounds. Money management. How to use OT in wherever you are. Improve quality of facility."
- "Co-treat and really collaborate with my clients to identify goals. Use EBP to direct actions. Build friendships. Have fun. Establish/enhance a life-giving legacy in my community. Learn/use effective documentation (especially for explaining the process). Create a photo essay."
- "How to communicate well with a different culture. Learn as much as I can about their culture. Be well organized. Be able

to help them with their goals. Make the projects both meaningful to them and also myself."

- "I would like to learn . . . confidence in self to help others and
  the ability to actively grade activities in a real-life setting. I
  am, however, looking forward to building relationships and
  learning community resources."
- "Appropriate way to communicate with a different population. Being assertive and confident in my position in the
  community so I can truly help the members."

Other reflection examples utilized through this service-learning
course included case studies, structured journals, group journals,
portfolio, small group discussions, interviews, role-playing, program
development, photo collections, presentations and celebrations at
the end of their service, and finally their article for publication. Each
group purchased a camera and documented their experiences with
photos and captions of reflections. These were also shared with the
community participants to aide in group reflection.

Intentionally linking the assessment of student learning outcomes
of service-learning with reflection is important and was completed
during this course. The following are two examples of student evaluations (Tables 6-6 and 6-7). The first example (Table 6-6) was given
pre- and post-experience with the students.

For the evaluation in Table 6-6, students averaged 3.89 at the beginning of the course and 4.56 at the completion of the course. For
the evaluation in Table 6-7, students averaged 4.67 following the
completion of the course.

The following are sample student reflections and comments on
the course:

- "This program has helped me a lot with the challenging
  health issues that we encounter. It is nice to get some information from other students and see what worked for them,
  and then take that and the other things we learn and go and
  try to change unhealthy behaviors. It makes all of the studying and work worthwhile when a client that we serve realizes
  that he has healthy alternatives to the food he eats, and that

Table 6-6 Student Evaluation of Service-Learning in a Course.

Please circle your response, using the following scale:

1 = Strongly Disagree   2 = Disagree   3 = Neutral   4 = Agree   5 = Strongly Agree

I feel comfortable working with individuals who are different from me (for example, age and ethnicity).	1	2	3	4	5
I feel knowledgeable about service-learning.	1	2	3	4	5
Being involved in my community is important to me.	1	2	3	4	5
I believe a service-learning course can make a positive contribution to the community.	1	2	3	4	5
I have a great understanding and appreciation for diversity.	1	2	3	4	5
Social problems are complex.	1	2	3	4	5
I feel culturally competent.	1	2	3	4	5
I feel comfortable with my interpersonal skills when working with someone different than me.	1	2	3	4	5
I learn more when I do service-learning in a course.	1	2	3	4	5
Service-learning makes me reflect on the importance of helping others.	1	2	3	4	5

Source: This survey was created by Dr. Callie Watson and Dr. Kristin Haas.

these choices can dramatically impact his health. I wouldn't have learned how to work with a patient on this if I weren't in this class."

- "The women at the care center are different from me. I am not accustomed to this 'culture.' Because of this, I learned I must think on my feet. This opportunity has helped me to analyze a different culture. The women are from quite diverse backgrounds having, broken families, live in a state of poverty, and have experienced things that I cannot even imagine.

Table 6-7 Student Evaluation Form of Service-Learning in a Course.

Please circle your response, using the following scale:
1 = Strongly Disagree 2 = Disagree 3 = Neutral 4 = Agree 5 = Strongly Agree

Sufficient class time was spent preparing me for my work in the community.	1	2	3	4	5
Sufficient training and supervision was provided by the agency.	1	2	3	4	5
The service work I performed helped me to learn the course content.	1	2	3	4	5
The reflection and analysis of my service in the course enhanced my learning.	1	2	3	4	5
I believe my service-learning made a positive contribution to the community.	1	2	3	4	5
The service-learning in the course has made me more likely to be active in the communities in which I live in the near future.	1	2	3	4	5
I have a greater appreciation for diversity as a result of my service-learning in this class.	1	2	3	4	5
Social problems are more complex than I used to think.	1	2	3	4	5
Service-learning in this class has helped me to develop my cultural competence.	1	2	3	4	5

Source: Courtesy of Kristin Mattson of Methodist College and Jennifer Reed-Bouley of College of St. Mary.

The longer I am at WCCH, the more I realize what a privilege money is, where money can get you, and what being a part of the right neighborhood and school and family can have on you."

- "I have never thought of myself as being naïve about social issues such as race and social class, but I am beginning to realize that I had just scratched the surface with my knowledge base. I hope to take this opportunity to expand my understanding of the socioeconomic situations in the United States and use my skills to help close the gap."

Reflections from Community Agencies

Faculty and students frequently are encouraged to reflect and to evaluate how the program is going. At CSM, we strive to maintain positive, long-lasting relationships with our community partners. Having the community agency participants and leaders reflect helps us to ensure that we are meeting our mission and objectives. Table 6-8 is an example of a survey developed to enable our community partners to reflect on the completed service-learning project.

Table 6-8 Community Partner Evaluation of Service-Learning in a Course.

1. The partnership with CSM was beneficial.

   Yes   No   Sometimes   Unsure

2. Students demonstrated professional behaviors at all times (i.e., showing up on time, respectful of staff time, wearing appropriate clothing, communicating appropriately, etc.).

   Always   Sometimes   Rarely   Not at all

3. Concerning the students, did they:

   Meet your expectations   Exceed expectations   Disappointed you

4. Will you use the resources provided by the students?

   Yes, all of them   Yes, some of them   Yes, a little   No, not at all   Unsure

5. What were some of the outcomes for you and your facility? What do you foresee as the outcomes in the future (if different)?

6. What did you like best?

7. What did you like least?

8. What could have made this experience better?

9. Would you want to work with CSM students, faculty and staff again?

   Yes   No   May be/Depends   Unsure

10. Comments:

Suggestions:

The following are a sampling of reflections from our community partners, both agency staff and program participants:

- "The students from CSM have made me realize that I can get out there and get a job and make it on my own. They are empowering and motivating."
- "The information on life skills was beneficial as many of us have never even applied or interviewed for a job. I look forward to seeing the students and having them practice on us."
- "This video and resource binder have changed things dramatically and have already reached hundreds of individuals, families, and groups. When the video is viewed it depicts the center exactly and puts things into perspective."
- "The video is touching, powerful, and will take us into the future. The partnership will continue to acquaint our residents with opportunities in education, community, and become overall healthier women who feel more connected to their community."

Faculty were also asked to reflect on the service-learning experience. Table 6-9 is a sample evaluation form for faculty to reflect on their service-learning experience.

Table 6-10 presents some reflections and comments gathered from faculty regarding the service-learning component of the course.

Table 6-9 Sample Faculty Evaluation Form of Service-Learning Experience.

1. What went well about this course?
2. What would you have liked to happen differently?
3. Do you believe the service-learning experience enhanced students' understanding of course content?
4. Do you believe the service-learning provided a benefit to the community agency and community in general?
5. Would you teach this class the same way again?

Source: Courtesy of Kristin Mattson of Methodist College and Jennifer Reed-Bouley of College of St. Mary.

Table 6-10 Faculty Reflections and Comments.

Lessons Learned

Volunteer and do favors for community partner/setting.

Have the relationship be ongoing.

Leave resources that can stay for a long time.

Do not just provide a service and leave.

Meet often with the community partner to be sure everyone understands expectations to avoid disappointment on either end.

Communication is key.

Helpful to pick agencies that share a common vision or mission.

Be sensitive to needs that may not be exactly what you had in mind.

Outcomes: Student, community partner, and/or faculty.

Closer bonds with students when doing service-learning.

Classes with service-learning stick out in mind more than others.

Learn students' true perceptions of socialcultural aspects.

Flexibility and understanding of nonprofit organizations.

Learn the power of doing favors for nonprofits.

Faculty: Shift to facilitator and advisor.

Trust the students are doing all they should be doing.

Personal growth and development from students.

See empowerment in students in getting more responsibility, being trusted, and providing a service that is needed and appreciated.

Moral development in students.

Higher self-esteem in students.

Students able to better recognize their strengths and assets.

See students struggle with now taking stronger responsibilities for their own learning.

See higher critical-thinking and problem-solving skills in students.

Students are better able to see the bigger picture.

See better outcomes with objectives in service-learning courses versus non–service-learning courses.

See collaboration and leadership roles come out in students that were "shy" in past.

See willingness to "take risks" in students and faculty.

See creativeness and improved communication skills and insight.

True understanding and appreciation of diversity in every sense of the word.

Higher motivation to complete projects for school and assignments.

Team work and group dynamics put into action (collaboration).

Networking is an outcome from service-learning.

CONCLUSION

Faculty at CSM provided an innovative approach towards teaching occupational therapy students competencies in health promotion in unique practice settings. The faculty at CSM have found that by bringing service-learning into the course work, students often perform at higher levels, attend class more, learn better problem solving and clinical thinking skills, feel class is more enjoyable, learn the true value of serving, and are more motivation to succeed. Students and faculty have formed bonds and presented both locally and nationally at conferences both inside and outside of the profession.

REFERENCES

American Occupational Therapy Association (AOTA). (2002). Occupational therapy practice framework: Domain and process. *American Journal of Occupational Therapy, 56*, 607.

Ash, S. L., Clayton, P. H., & Atkinson, M. P. (2005). Integrating reflection and assessment to capture and improve student learning. *Michigan Journal of Community Service-Learning, 11*(2), 49–60.

Astin, A., Vogelgesang, L., Ikeda, E., & Yee, J. (2000). *How service learning affects students.* Los Angeles: Higher Education Research Institute.

Astin, A. W., & Sax, L. J. (1998). How undergraduates are affected by service participation. *Journal of College Student Development, 39*(3), 251–263.

Balazadeh, N. (1996, October). *Service-learning and the sociological imagination: Approach and assessment.* Paper presented at the National Historically Black Colleges and Universities Faculty Development Symposium, Memphis, TN.

Berson, J. S., & Younkin, W. F. (1998, November). *Doing well by doing good: A study of the effects of a service-learning experience on student success.* Paper presented at the American Society of Higher Education Conference, Miami, FL.

Billig, S. (2006). Lessons from research on teaching and learning: Service-learning as effective instruction. In J. C. Kielsmeier, M. Neal, & A. Crossley (Eds.), *Growing to greatness 2006: The state of service learning* (pp. 25–32). Saint Paul, MN: National Youth Leadership Council.

Calleson, D. C., Parker, L., & Morgan, L. (1996). Institutional support for service-learning. *Journal of Research and Development in Education 31,* 147–154.

Clarke, M. M. (2000). Evaluating the Community Impact of Service Initiatives: The 3-I Model. *Unpublished Dissertation,* Nashville, TN: Peabody College, Vanderbilt University.

Cohen, J., & Kinsey, D. F. (1994). Doing good and scholarship: A service-learning study. *Journalism Educator, 48*(4), 4–14.

Driscoll, A., Holland, B., Gelmon, S., & Kerrigan, S. (1996). An assessment model for service-learning: Comprehensive case studies of impact on faculty, students, community, and institution. *Michigan Journal of Community Service Learning, 5,* 66–71.

Eyler, J., Giles, D., Stenson, C., & Gray, C. (2001). *At a glance: What we know about the effects of service-learning on college students, faculty, institutions and communities, 1993–2000,* 3rd edition. Learn and Serve America National Service-Learning Clearinghouse.

Eyler, J. S., & Giles, D. E. Jr. (1999). *Where's the learning in service-learning?* San Francisco: Jossey-Bass.

Ikeda, E. K. (1999). *How does service enhance learning? Toward an understanding of the process.* Unpublished doctoral dissertation, University of California, Los Angeles.

Kelly, P. J., Sylvia, E., Schwartz, l., Kuckelman Cobb, A., & Veal, K. (2006). Cameras and Community Health. *Journal of Psychosocial Nursing and Mental Health Services, 44,* 31–36.

McCawley, P. F. (2008). What is the logic model? University of Idaho Extension. Retrieved January 12, 2008, from http://www.uidaho.edu/extension/LogicModel.pdf.

Millar, A., Simeone, R. S., & Carnevale, J. T. (2001). Logic models: A systems tool for performance management. *Evaluation and Program Planning, 24,* 73–81.

Minkler, M. (1997). *Community organizing and community building for health.* Rutgers, NJ: Rutgers University Press.

Moon, J. (1999). *Reflection in learning and professional development.* London: Kogan Page Limited, Stylus Publishing Inc.

National Association of State Universities and Land Grant Colleges (1995). Retrieved May 12, 2008, from http://www.adec.edu/resources.

Pew Health Professions Commission. (1998). A joint report of the Pew Health Professions Commission and the Center for the Health Professions. University of California: San Francisco. Retrieved February 21, 2008, from http://www.futurehealth.ucsf.edu/compubs.html.

RMC Research. (2006/2008). Character education and service-learning. Scotts Valley, CA: National Service-Learning Clearinghouse. Retrieved April 1, 2008, from http://servicelearning.org/instant_info/fact_sheets/cb_facts/char_ed/index.php.

Sisters of Mercy. (2008). Retrieved March 21, 2008, from http://www.sistersofmercy.org/index.php?.

Stanton, T. (1994). The experience of faculty participants in an instructional development seminar on service-learning. *Michigan Journal of Community, 1*(1), 7–20.

Ward, S. (2000). Service-learning. *American Behavioral Scientist, 43*(5), 767–780.

Ward, K., & Vernon, A. (1999). *Community Perspectives on Student Volunteerism and Service Learning.* Paper presented at the 24th Annual Meeting of the Association for the Study of Higher Education, San Antonio, TX.

Western Washington University. (1994). Institutionalizing service learning in higher education. *Western Journal of Medicine, 168*(5), 400–411.

World Health Organization. (2008). Retrieved June 18, 2008, from http://www.who.int/en/.

World Health Organization. (2001). International Classification of Functioning, Disability, and Health (ICF). Geneva: Author.

World Health Organization. (1947). Constitution of the World Health Organization. New York: World Health Organization.

Course Syllabi and Forms

COLLEGE OF SAINT MARY
Health Promotion
OTH 417
Course Syllabus

CATALOG DESCRIPTION

This course examines the link between health, prevention of health problems, increased life satisfaction, and behavior patterns and lifestyles. The role of the occupational therapist as an educator is investigated and skills in patient education are developed. Emphasis is placed on the role of the occupational therapist in wellness prevention and healthy lifestyles. The OT's focus is purposeful and meaningful occupations; balance of rest, work, and play; and healthy interaction with the environment.

RELATIONSHIP TO CURRICULUM DESIGN

This course assists in preparing the student for graduate level work by instilling the role of an occupational therapist as an educator of consumers. Relevant health promotion and education techniques will be applied in future fieldwork experiences.

COURSE OBJECTIVES

Upon completion of this course, the student will be able to:

1. Employ logical thinking, critical analysis, problem solving, and creativity in health promotion and patient education.
2. Develop a holistic concept of health.
3. Compose a short publicity article related to OT's role in health promotion.
4. Demonstrate knowledge and appreciation of the role of sociocultural, socioeconomic, diversity factors, and lifestyles choices in contemporary society.
5. Appraise the influence of social conditions and the ethical context in which humans choose to engage in occupations.
6. Articulate to the consumer, potential employers, and the general public both the unique nature of occupation as viewed by the profession of occupational therapy and the value of occupation for the client.
7. Promote importance of the balance of performance areas to the achievement of health and wellness.
8. Pursue the role of occupation in the promotion of health and the prevention of disease and disability for the individual, family and society.
9. Evaluate the effects of health, disability, disease processes, and traumatic injury to the individual within the context of family and society.
10. Weigh the individual's perception of quality of life, well being, and occupation to promote health and prevent injury or disease.

TEACHING/LEARNING EXPERIENCES

Information will be provided through readings in assigned text and lectures.

The student is expected to:

1. Complete assigned reading prior to class.
2. Attend class on a regular basis.
3. Contribute *actively* toward expansion of learning experience through independent questioning, group discussions and participation in class assignments.
4. Use previous texts as supplemental references.
5. Incorporate principles learned in previous coursework into class activities.

SPECIFIC TEACHING/LEARNING METHODS THAT MAY BE USED

- Small group activity/presentations
- Guest lecture
- Case studies/intervention planning
- Audiovisual: slides, video, overhead
- Demonstration and practice
- Service-learning

Class Discussions/Facilitation	50 points
Article for Publication	150 points
Health Promotion Project	300 points
Grant Report	100 points
Peer Evaluations	50 points
Total:	**650 points**

DECLARATION OF OPEN DISCOURSE

In the spirit of intellectual inquiry, College of Saint Mary is committed to the exchange of diverse ideas and viewpoints. In this environment honest discourse is valued, demeaning remarks are not tolerated. Each member of the campus community is encouraged to:

- Recognize the basis of her or his own assumptions and perspectives,
- Acknowledge the assumptions and perspectives of others,
- Promote understanding and respectful dissent.

ASSIGNMENTS

Published Article

Compose a short publicity article related to OT's role in health pro-motion and/or concerning your project. Students must try to get this article published. Grading rubric given in class. (150 points)

Health Promotion Program/Project

Needs Analysis	50 points
Project	100 points
Communication with group and instructors	50 points
Presentation (in-service)	50 points
Peer Evaluations	50 points
Total:	**300 points**

Needs Analysis

A. Overview of the Facility: Provide a detailed description of the clients the facility it serves, location, space availability etc. (5 points)
B. How long has the facility been in existence? How is it funded? Where is it located and why? What is its mission? How is it meet-ing its mission? What programs are currently offered? Who is offering them? (5 points)
C. Program Development: Provide a brief statement as to the need of a program at this facility. What if any research is there to jus-tify such a program? (10 points)
D. SWOT Analysis: Complete a SWOT analysis ON THIS PROGRAM/ PROJECT (10 points):
   1. What are the strengths of the facility (internal)?
   2. What are its weaknesses (internal)?
   3. What are opportunities for the facility (external)?
   4. What are potential threats for the facility (external)?

E. Program Goals: What are your goals for your program? Include specific time frames. Are your time frames realistic? How will you know if you met your goals? Who will run this program? (5 points)
F. Strategies: What are the specific strategies used to meet each of your identified goals? Include time frames and who is responsible for meeting the goals. (5 points)
G. Program Evaluation: How will you monitor if your program is effective? How often will you evaluate your program? Who will complete the data collection and how will they store the data? (5 points)
H. References (APA format) (5 points)

Project

Organization	20 points
Neatness (grammar/spelling)	15 points
Creativity	10 points
Research component (also utilizing needs analysis information)	30 points
Program meets needs (facility evaluation)	25 points
	100 points

Communication with Group and Instructors

It is imperative to keep all classmates and instructors up-to-date with current project. Students are expected to cc group members and instructors on all e-mail correspondence. Instructors must get an update weekly either by phone, e-mail or face to face interaction regarding project/service-learning.

Correspondence was appropriate and professional (no spelling errors, etc.)	10 points
Correspondence was timely (met all deadlines)	40 points
	50 points

Presentation

Professional presentation and appearance	5 points
Logical selection of pertinent information	10 points
Creativity of presentation	10 points
Knowledge of proposal	25 points
	50 points

Grant Report

Overview	20 points
Budget	40 points
Social Analysis and Critical Reflection/ Reflection Outcomes	20 points
Evaluation	20 points
	100 points

Class Discussions/Assignments

This course helps to prepare students for graduate level work. At graduate level, we expect students to not only report facts but interpret classroom information and present new information or describe application of knowledge. Please note this course is to permit you to question and think critically about topics that may or may not be new to you. Participation (in this course and graduate level courses) is vital. It is expected for students to present material in a professional manner, participate in dialogue, to ask questions and search for answers (on own). This also means students are expected to bring in outside resources to enhance the richness of classroom participation.

In this course, you will be representing College of Saint Mary at various community settings (see service learning information at end of syllabus for further instruction). Students are expected to be professional at all times. Students are encouraged to show initiative and self directed learning (beyond the classroom). At sometime during the course, the instructor will be providing feedback regarding performance inside and outside of the classroom. If a student experiences any difficulties, does not feel as though they are being treated respectfully (either by faculty or peers), or has any grievances for the instructor (or course), it is the responsibility of the student to make an appointment immediately with the instructor.

> 30 points (total): Asks questions almost every class, depth and breadth of material presented, brings in outside resources almost every class.
>
> 25 points: Discusses topics well, but only hits surface of material, brings in one outside resource and asks only five questions throughout semester.
>
> 20 points: Asks only a few questions, minimally participants with discussion, and does not bring in outside resources.

Class facilitation	20 points
In-class assignments and participation	30 points
	50 points

STATEMENT OF PROFESSIONAL BEHAVIOR

Inherent in the profession of occupational therapy, there are values that are demonstrated through professional behavior. Examples of professional behavior include, but are not limited to: being dependable, demonstrating collaboration and cooperation, exhibiting initiative and appropriate communication skills, sensitivity toward the feelings and behaviors of others, accepting and modifying performance based on meaningful feedback, learning appropriate written communication skills and exhibiting professional verbal communication skills with others such as sharing and being constructive.

TOPICAL OUTLINE

DATE	TOPIC	ASSIGNMENT
Jan 15	Introduction to Course and Syllabus APA and Writing Service-Learning Needs Analysis Grant/Budget Level I D Fieldwork Assignment	Discussion of publishing articles and ideas (examples)* Discussion of service-learning, expectations and projects in course* Discussion of needs analysis*
Jan 22	What is Health? Health Promotion Across the Lifespan: Older Adults and Women Needs Analysis Continued	**Project Placement Decision Due**
Jan 29	**Field trips** Mercy Housing: Mason Apts WCCH Ollie Webb Morton Magnet Middle School	**Please plan to get out for lunch with classmates and faculty**
Feb 5	Health Promotion Across the Lifespan: Men and Youth Stress Management	
Feb 12	Promoting the Health of Communities Using the OT approach for health promotion, consultation and networking Articles on health promotion	
Feb 19	Community Setting	Time for Assignments
Feb 26	Community Setting	Time for Assignments
Mar 4	**No Class: Spring Break**	**Enjoy Spring Break**
Mar 11	Community Setting	Time for Assignments
Mar 18	Community Setting	Time for Assignments

Mar 25	Community Setting	**Article Draft Due**
		Must meet with instructors one on one for advising of articles
April 1	Community Setting	Time for Assignments
		Project Draft Due
April 8	Community Setting	Time for Assignments
		Articles should be submitted for publication by now
		Grant Report Draft Due
April 15	Community Setting	Time for Assignments
April 22– May 16	**Project Celebration/ Presentation**	**Final Article Due**
	Wrap Up	

*Instructor(s) facilitates class instruction.
**Please note syllabus is subject to change (especially due to community settings).

SERVICE-LEARNING IN OTH 417

This course is an intensive community/experientially based learning course. Research suggests there are many personal and social outcomes to service learning (see handout to be distributed in class for specific resources). Students are expected to observe, participate, and reflect/analyze through discussion, writing, video, and/or presentations in order to integrate course content to real-life experience. Students are expected to adhere to the OT student manual regarding professionalism and professional dress for community settings.

Service learning includes the following and will be discussed in further detail in class:

Reciprocal benefits
Deliberate reflection
Community identified needs

Partnership
Process as central
Power is shared
More than just volunteering time

REFLECTIONS/OUTCOMES ON EXPERIENCE

Today I learned . . .

Today, what did you learn to demonstrate knowledge and appreciation of the role of sociocultural, socioeconomic, diversity factors, and lifestyles choices in contemporary society?

Today, what did you learn to appraise the influence of social conditions and the ethical context in which humans choose to engage in occupations?

Comment on whether you think the participants at your community agency are more likely to eat healthier.

Reflect on how you were or were not able to help the participants at your community agency to increase their self concept and develop self-advocacy skills.

Comment on the following statement:
I learned the value to serve (through this course).

Comment on the following statements:
This course helped to promote critical thinking.
This experience helped me to analyze the social dimensions and contexts (including such issues as race, social class and gender).

List three things I learned today (i.e., mission, facts, issues in community, etc.)

Why is service-learning important?

What will you do with your new knowledge, personally and professionally?

Overall this experience has taught me. . .

This experience has impacted me positively by. . .

This experience has impacted me negatively by. . .

Please add any comments that will help for future participants.

PEER/SELF GROUP INTERACTION ASSESSMENT

Please evaluate **each** member of your group **and yourself**. You are expected to evaluate each member/self **honestly**. Please record your evaluation responses below their names. Please e-mail to the instructor as soon as you have completed them. It is encouraged that you take notes throughout the learning process to help give examples and constructive feedback for your classmates. Be assured that your confidentiality will be maintained. You will be graded on how well you assess and give feedback to your classmates. If you feel you need guidance in making comments constructive, please see instructor immediately.

Your name: _____

Student's name you are evaluating: _____

Please indicate your response using the following rating guide:

- 5 = Student is consistent and provides excellent contributions
- 4 = Student is generally consistent and provides very good contributions
- 3 = Student is somewhat consistent and provides satisfactory contributions
- 2 = Student is somewhat inconsistent and provides unsatisfactory contributions
- 1 = Student is inconsistent and provides inappropriate contributions (or doesn't contribute at all)

Overall rating for this student (see scale above, rate from 5–1) _____

Assessment Items	Yes, No, Sometimes	Comments
1. This person actively contributes to group discussions.		
2. This person came prepared for class.		
3. This person helps to redirect discussions when the group gets "off track."		
4. This person listens to the opinions and contributions of others.		
5. This person exercises mutual respect for others in the group.		
6. This person helps keep the group focused on the timeline.		
7. This person works well with the other group members.		
8. This person does not monopolize group discussions.		
9. This person performs assigned tasks in group well.		
10. This person shares their knowledge within the group.		

Additional Comments:

Morton Middle School Course Syllabus
CSM Presents Morton I.D.O.L.S.
Morton Magnet Middle School
Be Responsible, Be Respectful, Be Safe.
Instructors: Cathy Buchmeier, Sunee Haney, Kari Koster, and Sara Mashek
College of Saint Mary Occupational Therapy Students

Class Day/Time: Friday, 1:09 p.m.–2:39 p.m.
Class Description: This class examines the link between health and prevention of health problems, increased life satisfaction, behavior patterns, and lifestyles. Student's focus should be on balance of rest, work, play, and healthy interaction with the environment.
Semester Schedule:

Date	Instructors	Class Topic
Feb 22	Cathy, Kari, Sara, & Sunee	Hobbies & Leisure
Feb 29	Cathy & Sunee	Exercise
Mar 7	Cathy	TBA*
Mar 14	Cathy & Sunee	Art
Mar 21	Ms Rodriguez	TBA*
Mar 28	Sara & Sunee	Women's Health
Apr 4	Kari & Sara	Self-Defense
Apr 18	Kari, Sara, Sunee, & Cathy	Field Trip!!
Apr 25	Sunee & Cathy	Service Learning (field trip)
May 2	Kari & Cathy	Healthy Eating
May 9	Kari & Sara	Relationships
May 16	Ms Rodriguez	TBA*

*To be announced.

Student Expectations

	Criteria				Points
	4	3	2	1	
Attendance/ Promptness	Student is always prompt and regularly attends classes.	Student is late to class once every two weeks and regularly attends classes.	Student is late to class more than once every two weeks and regularly attends classes.	Student is late to class more than once a week and/or has poor attendance of classes.	____
Level of Engagement in Class	Student proactively contributes to class by offering ideas and asking questions more than once per class.	Student proactively contributes to class by offering ideas and asking questions once per class.	Student rarely contributes to class by offering ideas and asking questions.	Student never contributes to class by offering ideas and asking questions.	____

(continued)

(*Continued*)

Listening Skills	Student listens when others talk, both in groups and in class. Student incorporates or builds off of the ideas of others.	Student listens when others talk, both in groups and in class.	Student does not listen when others talk, both in groups and in class.	Student does not listen when others talk, both in groups and in class. Student often interrupts when others speak.	____
Behavior	Student almost never displays disruptive behavior during class.	Student rarely displays disruptive behavior during class.	Student occasionally displays disruptive behavior during class.	Student almost always displays disruptive behavior during class.	____
Preparation	Student is almost always prepared for class with assignments and required class materials.	Student is usually prepared for class with assignments and required class materials.	Student is rarely prepared for class with assignments and required class materials.	Student is almost never prepared for class with assignments and required class materials.	____
				Total	____

Teacher Comments:

SAMPLE CLASS OUTLINES FOR OLLIE WEBB CENTER

April 1st

- 6–6:05 Welcome group members
- 6:05–6:20 Talk about occupational therapy

- 6:20–7:00 Split up into groups and make their designated food items (As groups get done we will have activities for them to do while they wait.)
- 7–7:30 Eat the food
- 7:30–7:50 Reflect on how making the food went and what they thought was hard or easy about cooking.
- 7:50–8:00 Say goodbye and give them a note for next class. Class celebration at bowling alley.

April 8

- 6–6:15 Arrive at the bowling alley
- 6:15–6:25 Get shoes and lanes
- 6:25–7:30 Bowl
- 7:30–7:45 Give shoes back
- 7:45–8:00 Give them their picture books and thank them for participating in our group
- Reflect and discuss hobbies, sports, and health

MASON OBJECTIVES FOR COLLABORATING WITH THE WOMEN OF MASON

1. Promote health by learning and participating in relaxation techniques through the practice of yoga.
2. Promote health by providing a client-centered resource to utilize on an on-going basis.
3. Promote health by raising awareness of factors influencing personal wellness.
4. Verify interests of the women regarding activities of wellness.
5. Understand the perspective of "healthy" among women from another culture.
   a. What does it look like to be healthy?

DATES AND TIMES OF SESSIONS

- Monday, March 31, from 10 am–Noon
- Tuesday, April 1, from 10 am–Noon
- Monday, April 7, from 10 am–Noon
- Thursday, April 10, from 10 am–Noon

Promote health by learning and participating in relaxation techniques through the practice of yoga.

- In order to promote health, women will learn and participate in 1–4 yoga sessions of 30–60 minutes. Each of the four sessions will include 30–45 minutes of practicing yoga and learning relaxation techniques. Each session will be held in the Network Center (unless space requires us to move into the hall upstairs). If the women are interested in continuing yoga, yoga mats may be purchased. Provide nametags and healthy snacks for each session and translating is available.

Promote health by providing a client-centered resource to utilize on an ongoing basis.

- In order to promote health, women will be provided with a client-centered resource to address primary health concerns, while taking into account the need for pictures as the sole "language" of the resource. Health concerns will be identified in the first session, Monday, March 31, via a survey/discussion.

Promote health by raising awareness of factors influencing personal wellness.

- In order to promote health, women will raise their own awareness of factors influencing their health by completing a short survey on, Monday, March 31.

Verify interests of the women regarding activities of wellness.

- In order to promote client-centered health, women will verify personal activities of wellness she uses or wants to use by completing a short survey Monday, March 31.

Understand the perspective of "healthy" among women from another culture.

- In order to promote health, women will photograph people, places, or things that answer one of the two questions, *What does "healthy" look like?* or *What does "unhealthy" look like?* This type of project using photography is modified from a previously established approach called *Photovoice* (Kelly, Sylvia, Schwartz, Kuckelman, & Veal, 2006). It aids in empowering individuals and in helping develop their voice.
- Women will photograph 27 images within one week to answer the above question. Women will be given the cameras, instructions, and objectives Tuesday, April 1.
  - Objectives of Photovoice:
    - Identify images of health
    - Identify personal beliefs of health in order to further inspire health and to be able to provide individuals from other cultures a more sincere view of the meaning for these women of "health" to be able to better provide client-centered options.
- Monday, April 7, women will turn in their cameras. An additional and client-centered activity will be added here, pending the information provided. from the surveys.
- Tuesday, April 10, women will receive their developed photographs. Each participant will choose 3–4 photographs she likes, then discuss them/answer questions such as:
  - What did you see?
  - What's really happening in this image?
  - How does what's happening in the picture relate to health?
  - Why does this image portray health?
  - How might we use what we've seen in and learned from this image to better address our own health?
  - What can we do about the health of the women of Mason? As individuals? As a group?
- Each participant will then choose their favorite image of health. This image will be framed, delivered to the individual, and potentially hung in a "showing."
- Lastly, each participant will complete a questionnaire about what being in the project meant to them and what she can do to influence her own health.

Mission Statements

College of Saint Mary Mission

Committed to the works, values and aspirations of the Sisters of Mercy, College of Saint Mary is a Catholic college dedicated to the education of women in an environment that calls forth potential and fosters leadership. This mission inspires us to:

- Academic excellence, scholarship, and lifelong learning
- Regard for the dignity of each person
- Attention to the development of mind, body, and spirit
- Compassionate service to others

College of Saint Mary Occupational Therapy Mission

The Occupational Therapy Program at the College of Saint Mary strives to provide a high quality educational environment and foster academic excellence and leadership among women. Graduates become occupational therapists who are prepared to integrate the spirit with the mind and body through occupation. The program prepares students to deliver quality occupational therapy services and respond to fluctuations in the overall health care system.

Graduates of the program are equipped with the knowledge and skills to promote quality of life that is expressed in meaningful doing or occupation. The Occupational Therapy Program emphasizes providing compassionate, ethical occupational therapy services to all individuals, particularly those who are vulnerable to compromised health and quality living.

Chapter 7

Occupation of Learning Through Service Engagement: An Occupational Therapy Assistant Program Perspective

Diane Sauter-Davis, MA, OTR/L

Service and community engagement are essential aspects of professional formation of occupational therapy assistants at Kennebec Valley Community College (KVCC). This chapter provides an overview of the context of service-learning at this institution and specifically within the occupational therapy assistant (OTA) program. Additionally, it provides ideas and techniques for developing learning through community engagement in any occupational therapy program.

KVCC is committed to service-learning through its Center for Civic Engagement (CCE). The center was established through the passion and vision of the college president. Starting with VISTA volunteers and a small group of committed faculty members, service-learning is now integrated into many courses and programs at the college.

In 2000, the CCE initiated faculty involvement under the volunteer direction of the Humanities department chair. Faculty members were invited by the Humanities department chair to participate in developing service-learning within the context of their courses. Faculty members were also supported to participate in national service-learning coalitions, such as Campus Compact: National Center for Community Colleges. Eventually, a mentoring program developed by faculty for faculty provided support to those interested in incorporating service-learning into their courses. A *KVCC Faculty Service Learning Handbook* (*KVCC, FSLH*), created by this core group of mentors was provided to all faculty. This handbook provided the philosophy of service-learning at KVCC and the varied definitions of service-learning. It provided examples of excellence and templates to build service-learning experiences in a variety of coursework. A *Student Service Learning Handbook* (*KVCC, SSLH*) and database were also developed to support students with guidelines and community sites to enhance service-learning endeavors.

INSTITUTIONAL SUPPORT

The Center for Civic Engagement (CCE) was created to provide an official structure for the institutionalization of service-learning at KVCC. The major goals of the CCE are to:

- Promote the development of service-learning courses
- Provide education and consultation to faculty interested in developing service-learning courses
- Promote and support a high degree of community involvement and civic engagement across all aspects of the campus community

- Develop and maintain a library of reference materials on service-learning and civic engagement
- Track the service and volunteer hours of the campus community
- Develop and maintain a database and communication structure between the campus and community partners
- Assist students who are engaged in service to create "links" between academic and real-world learning
- Provide students with experiences to enhance their knowledge of diversity within our community (*KVCC, SSLH,* p. 1)

The value of institutional support cannot be overstated; it is essential to the subsequent acceptance of service-learning pedagogy (Hinck & Brandell, 2000). Institutional support is the genesis of this acceptance. It was an institutional leader, the Humanities chair (the CCE director) who began building momentum for the KVCC service-learning experience. The chair created and compiled resources from lists of involved community partners and designed a database of these partners. This database was made available to students and faculty. Additionally, service-learning opportunities were posted on bulletin boards across campus and on the CCE Web page. Mentoring options for faculty interested in learning more about service-learning were described at faculty meetings. Finally, institutional support provided limited financial reimbursement for faculty to design, implement and evaluate service-learning experiences and courses.

SERVICE-LEARNING: THE OCCUPATIONAL THERAPY ASSISTANT PROGRAM

The Occupational Therapy Assistant (OTA) program at KVCC initiated-learning through community collaboration long before the college officially endorsed the value of service-learning through the development of the Center for Civic Engagement (CCE). This collaboration was consistent with our mission and philosophy of integrated learning and curriculum design (see Table 7-1).

Table 7-1 Mission and Philosophy of the OTA Program.

Mission	Philosophy
The mission of the OTA program is to prepare students to become competent Occupational Therapy Assistants who will provide Maine with a cadre of qualified and dedicated occupational therapy practitioners to assist its citizens in achieving independence and wellness while maintaining individual choice, human dignity and personal satisfaction.	The philosophy of our Occupational Therapy Assistant Program is consistent with the Philosophical Base of Occupational Therapy (1979) and the Philosophy of Occupational Therapy Education Statement (2003). The Philosophy of the OTA Program at KVCC is an integrated approach based on occupational therapy principles and the Model of Human Occupation. We also value the Quality of Life Framework and the practical guidance of John Dewey, educator and philosopher. Based on these foundations the OTA program thrives on the concepts of: • motivation, habituation, and performance; • participation and engagement in occupation; • integration and adaptation; • being, belonging, and becoming; and doing; • learning through experimentation; practice and feedback.

Source: Kennebec Valley Community College OTA Student Handbook (2009).

The initial service-learning course experiences were developed with the OTA Mental Health Concepts course in 1993. It was, and continues to be called, the Community Collaboration Project. This project arose out of the need to provide real life intervention situations for students while meeting community needs. The project engaged students to complete an environmental scan of their communities using needs assessment principles. Based on the needs and assets of the community, course learning objectives and community engagement activities were established with community partners. Reflection activities and competencies for assessment of student occupational therapy skills in community were put into operation in order to assess student learning and community outcomes.

Over time, we have collected course outcomes demonstrating that student engagement and real-time problem-solving opportunities coupled with guided client interfacing enhanced first year, second semester, student readiness for their fieldwork Level I learning experiences. Feedback from students about their service-learning experiences was very positive. Additionally, feedback from sites demonstrated that the students were meeting a community need, reinforcing the philosophy of service-learning regarding reciprocity for student learning and community enhancement.

Based on this feedback and the growth in student professional skills (i.e., observation, therapeutic use of self, intervention planning, and problem solving), we began to consider how this service engagement could be beneficial in other courses within the OTA program. We have subsequently incorporated service-learning experiences with two additional courses. Service-learning is now a primary learning tool in two core occupational therapy courses and a small component in another occupational therapy course. Service-learning has become an integral part of student learning in two general education courses within the OTA program.

Our role as occupational therapy educators is to assist students to solve problems creatively, negotiate the healthcare world successfully and to become competent, resourceful occupational therapy professionals. Studies and scholarly articles related to occupational therapy education using service-learning and community engagement demonstrate the value of these learning experiences to address these professional skills (Beck & Barnes, 2007). Student feedback from our coursework reflection and evaluation also suggests that through service-learning students have learned, and continue to learn, how to create something meaningful through participation and engagement and become competent and resourceful negotiators in the healthcare arena (Troppe, 1995).

Service-learning is a natural link toward integration of our pedagogical integrity as educators with our program's mission and philosophy (see Table 7-1). Schkade (1999) states, "the transition from classroom to clinic or other intervention settings is one of a series of professional transitions in the occupational role of practitioner" and "to achieve the desired outcome of emerging competence in occupational functioning, as a practitioner, the student must adapt to professional challenges that the workplace presents" (Schkade, 1999, p. 148). Service-learning provides a structure that can be used to promote and facilitate student competence.

The Deweyan notion of experiential learning calls for "authentic" forms of instruction and assessment wherein the student might more readily see, act on, and learn from connections between academic content and problems of real life (Strange, 2000). Dewey asserted that knowledge is the outcome of successful inquiry (McGreal, 1992). As defined by Kolbe (1996):

> . . . service learning is both a program type and a philosophy of education. As a program type, it includes myriad ways that students can perform meaningful service to their communities and to society while engaging in some form of reflection or study that is related to the service. As a philosophy of education, service-learning reflects the belief that education must be linked to social responsibility and that the most effective learning is active and connected to experience in some meaningful way. (Preface)

No matter which construct or definition is used, service-learning is action oriented, learning by doing; it is knowledge built through action. This philosophy directly supports our institution's mission "to prepare students to achieve their educational, professional, and personal goals in a supportive environment through shared values of responsibility, integrity, and respect" and vision for our graduates "to utilize their education and knowledge for productive and responsible citizenship" (Kennebec Community College, 2008, p. 4) as well as the Occupational Therapy Assistant program's mission and philosophy (Table 7-1). The positive input of service-learning for occupational therapy assistant students is notable regarding student learning outcomes. The long-term positive contributions of service-learning for future community participation and leadership have been well documented by Fenzel and Peyrot (2005).

SERVICE-LEARNING COURSES

The OTA courses that currently integrate service-learning are Occupational Therapy across the Lifespan I and Occupational Therapy across the Lifespan II. These courses are deeply rooted content related to occupational therapy theory and intervention techniques. Although both courses discuss service delivery across the lifespan; each course has a distinct focus. Lifespan I has a mental health focus; Lifespan II a developmental/physical disabilities core. Additionally, there is a service-learning link in our Interpersonal Skills for the Allied Health Professional course.

Service-learning in each of these courses has a definitive purpose related to the unique course learning objectives and methods. According to Zlotkowski (1998), linking the academic theory to the praxis allows for improved critical-reasoning skills, personal discovery of strengths and challenges, and experience and feedback to balance out theoretical knowledge. The inclusion of service-learning has been an effective teaching and learning strategy within each course and has become a key pedagogical tool for student understanding of key course learning objectives.

Occupational Therapy Across the Lifespan I

Service-learning is an integral part of the coursework in this five-credit class. It is still called the "Community Collaboration Project" (CCP), because this truly reflects the essence of the class. The CCP is mandatory, content driven, student initiated, and reflective. The foci for learning and reflection are on the psychosocial and behavior health needs of human beings. Service-learning counts for 20% of the total grade.

The purpose of the CCP is to apply classroom theory to OT practice in the field. In particular, observation, interview, documentation,

Table 7-2 Occupation of Learning Through Service Engagement: The Syllabi.

COURSE TITLE: Occupational Therapy Across the Lifespan I

COURSE DESCRIPTION: This course is the first of two lifespan courses. It provides students the opportunity to explore Occupational Therapy theory and practice, and the role of the OTA relative to behavioral health care. Major mental health diagnoses and the way in which they interfere with occupational performance across the lifespan will be examined. Students will explore systems of service delivery, models of service, and roles for occupational therapy assistants consistent with the current delivery of behavioral health services. Students learn to create occupation-based interventions based on activity analysis, critical thinking, and evidence. Participation, engagement and quality of life issues are examined. This course involves integrated lab experiences to support learning. Students will interact in the community through service learning projects relevant to OT psychosocial practice.

Pertinent Course Objectives relative to service-learning:

Upon completion of this course, the student should be able to:

- Define and demonstrate therapeutic use of self as a means of achieving therapeutic goals.
- Define and demonstrate an understanding of cultural competence.
- Recognize and demonstrate the importance of accurate documentation of services to ensure accountability of service provision and reimbursement standards.
- Explore the role of occupation in the promotion of wellness and the individual perspective of quality of life.
- Plan and implement individual and group treatment, using therapeutic use of self as a means of achieving goals.
- Demonstrate emerging professionalism in documentation skills typically exhibited by OTAs.
- Practice therapeutic use of self.
- Demonstrate effective collaborative relationships.

activity analysis, therapeutic use of self, goal setting, and time management skills are practiced (Table 7-2). Reflection is a key component.

Students receive a community experience assignment upon receiving the syllabus (Table 7-3). The assignment includes an overview, learning objectives, flexible timelines for completion, and requirements for time at the site. A final presentation is the capstone. All expectations are outlined, including that the focus for this learning is on mental

Table 7-3 Occupational Therapy Across the Lifespan I: Assignments and Grading.

I. Choose an environment (facility or individual is OK) in the community.

II. When choosing a setting, you must first:

    1. Contact the individual or the director of the facility you are interested in. If you need a letter of explanation, contact the Program Director.

    2. Set up a meeting with individual or facility to explain the assignment. Make sure to explain that you are not providing OT services but rather practicing the following skills by spending time with an individual/group that might benefit.

      • Interviewing

      • Understanding of psychosocial and behavioral issues

      • Communication

      • Observation

      • Documentation

      • Intervention planning/goal setting/outcome planning

      • Activity analysis/selection

      • Time management /professionalism

    3. Discuss with the person or the director of the facility that you hope to visit weekly for a minimum of 10 hours, cumulatively.

III. Write a letter of intent.

IV. Only after your intent is approved may you move forward with setting up appointment times with individual/facility.

V. Once you have gotten permission to work with a client(s) you will need to:

    1. Set up a regularly scheduled meeting time(s) at the facility.

    2. Write a note of explanation re: time descriptors (ex-1/week for 1 hour, terms of service learning, duties of your experience, etc.) You must keep a log of every visit.

    3. Document each visit using SOAP note format. One note is due for each visit for a total of 10. One note/each visit is required. No identifying information (HIPAA violation) is to be documented or disclosed. Each note should be handed in on the following Wednesday (i.e., if you do a visit on Friday then a note will be due on the *next* Wednesday).

    REMINDER: ANY confidentiality violation is grounds for immediate dismissal from the program.

    4. Interview the person(s) using forms from classes or books (i.e., activity configurations, interest checklists, COPM, role identification, etc.).

(continued)

Table 7-3 (*Continued*)

If you are doing general service at the facility, use these checklists to support your learning in general.

5. Find out what interests/goals the person(s) might have. Identify a goal and an activity you would like to complete with an individual/group or for the facility and include your rationale for this choice. (i.e., JB will attend 5 of 6 group trips in 6 weeks to increase interaction in the community to promote social participation. This is due after your fourth visit.)

6. Complete 10 meetings at the site by carrying out activities for 10 weeks. Write at least one page about your learning "success" and/or "failure," including rationale.

7. Your last session with the person/at the facility should involve a gesture of appreciation to both the person and the setting in recognition of their participation in your education.

8. Complete all other service-learning paper work as required.
   - One letter of intent
   - Evidence log of visits and times
   - One assessment/routine/functional goal-setting form
   - Five SOAP notes
   - List of activities completed and created
   - One "Before" Reflection Form; five "During" Reflection Forms, one "After" Reflection Form
   - Community Collaboration Reflection
   - Presentation PowerPoint with completed project binder
   - Work must be handed in at a regular pace. Work will be reviewed, feedback provided, and returned. Work will be graded as an aggregate and a check mark/date given. All check marked works must be compiled and handed in with PowerPoint presentation

VI. Final presentations will be for 10 minutes. Presentations will be in a case study format.

---

illness/behavior health across the lifespan. Students are asked to review expectations and develop an intent statement before beginning.

Students find their own site based on individual interest, geography, and experience. They are asked to take a risk with a population that is unfamiliar to them (e.g., if they have experience working with children, then they are asked to challenge themselves to work with adults). A faculty member is available to discuss their choices and options. Issues regarding safety are discussed. There is, for example, no transporting of persons while undertaking service-learning. Students begin to research their local communities. They contact the person/facility and explain the assignment and begin.

Reflection is crucial to our service-learning process. Reflection is the connecting piece; it is critical thinking in action. Student reflections are full of "ah ha" moments and are sometime the genesis for understanding the complexities of human beings within the healthcare system. We require three levels of reflection: before, during (ongoing), and after. Students are asked to complete a series of questions before they begin. These questions focus on guiding the student to reflect and connect theory to action.

Examples of before questions might include: What do you think your project or service site will be like?, How do you think this theory class will impact your learning and vice versa?, What issues do you think your project or the service site addresses?, What impact do you think you will have on the people you will be working for or with?, and How do you think OT could help?

Examples of during questions might include: What are you learning in class that supports/negates what you are seeing at your site?, What are the most difficult and enjoyable parts of this service activity? Why?, and What surprises you about what your reactions to the person/people at your site?

Examples of after service-learning questions might include: What have you learned from any disappointment or successes in your project?, What did you do that seemed to be effective or ineffective in your service-learning project?, How does your understanding of the value of occupation change as a result of your project?, and Was your understanding of the class work enhanced, magnified, or made more understandable as a result of your participation in this project?

Table 7-4 illustrates examples of lessons learned and course challenges that provide opportunities for students, faculty, and community partners to come together to find creative, collaborative strategies, and solutions for the dynamic learning and growth that can occur through community engagement experiences.

Table 7-4 Challenges and Solutions.

Challenges	Solutions
Students who cannot articulate the assignment and the objectives to sites are often turned down. This is a teachable moment, worthy of reflection and feedback.	Students are mentored in how to articulate the assignment. Individual strategies are discussed and practiced. Immediate feedback about professional presentation is available.
Students who are fearful to take the initiative and therefore do not begin in enough time to complete mindfully and/or successfully.	Class brainstorming, after the assignment is given, helps timid students to increase their comfort level and gain ideas. In some cases, a letter from the OTA program director outlining the service-learning activity is the best solution to help the student begin.
Students who are fearful of expectations, time demands, and assignments (including confidentiality and HIPAA regulations).	A well-developed outline helps to keep the expectations clear. Students are able to intertwine service-learning projects. This helps to manage time, but in this case the intent paper is very important. As part of the assignment students learn about HIPAA and sign a letter of attestation/confidentiality. This is presented to each individual/site.
Students do not know the difference between a reaction and a reflection.	Students must sometimes be coached on the difference between a reaction, and a reflection. All students are educated about the value of becoming a reflective practitionerand how reflection enhances critical thinking and clinical reasoning. In some cases, examples of reflection are given and practiced verbally.

Occupational Therapy Across the Lifespan II

Occupational Therapy across the Lifespan II is the sequential course to Occupational Therapy Across the Lifespan I. Currently, it is a 10-credit course with four population-focus modules: pediatrics, adults with developmental disabilities, adults with physical disabilities, and elders. This course is cotaught and modules overlap and interrelate. Service-learning is the practical anchor of the course (Table 7-5).

The purpose of the community engagement assignment is to apply classroom theory to occupational therapy practice in the field. In particular: observation, interview, documentation, activity analysis, therapeutic use of self, goal setting, and time management skills will be practiced. Specific content is addressed (i.e., use of assessment tools, fall prevention programming, environmental modification, assistive technology, safety education, etc.). Reflection remains a key component. Lab time is given to complete this activity. Service-learning "lab time" is unique to this process and does not compete with "in class" lab experiences.

Students receive the community engagement experience assignment upon receiving the syllabus. Again, the assignment includes: overview, learning objectives, flexible timelines for completion and requirements for time at site, and final presentation (Table 7-3). All expectations are outlined, including that the focus for this learning is on developmental disorders (children and adults), physical dysfunction, and or elder issues. Students may choose to find their own site based on interest, geography, and experience or they may choose a local site(s) that has expressed a specific service need. They may work independently or in teams or small groups. They are asked to take a risk with a population that is unfamiliar (e.g., if they have experience working with children, then challenge themselves to work with adults). A faculty member is available to discuss their choices and options. Again, safety is always reviewed. Students begin to research their local communities. They contact the person/facility to explain the assignment and begin.

The concept of reflection is more implicit during this second service-learning experience. Reflection assignments remain critical to student success. Students are asked to reflect using all of their cumulative knowledge, including that gained from the CCP. We make attempts to use group reflection in the classroom to better understand reflection and its place within the critical-thinking process. Use of group reflection has the potential to move internal thinking

Table 7-5 Occupation of Learning Through Service Engagement: The Syllabi.

COURSE TITLE: Occupational Therapy Across the Lifespan II

COURSE DESCRIPTION: This course provides students the opportunity to explore and understand Occupational Therapy practice relative to physical disabilities. Students will examine the stages of development and the impact of health, disease, injury, and disability on occupational performance and participation. This course will be taught in linking modules from infancy to eldercare. Emphasis in each module will be placed on the lifecycle issues and occupations, intervention techniques, service delivery systems, and policies relevant to the particular module focus. Quality of life is presented as an integral concept. This course involves integrated lab experiences that provide students opportunities to learn, practice, and demonstrate clinical skills. A service-learning lab is exclusive to the academic lab. An open mentor lab is included.

Pertinent Course Objectives relative to service-learning objectives:

Upon completion of this course the student will be able to:

- Identify and discuss various settings where children (0–20) receive OT services and the service delivery systems used in a child's natural environment.
- Discuss the role and function of the OTA in assessing and treating persons with physical disabilities and eldercare.
- Describe occupational therapy interventions that maximize occupational function in persons with physical impairments.
- Demonstrate the ability to interact through written, oral, and nonverbal communication.
- Recognize the importance for all healthcare workers to understand and follow safety policies and procedures.
- Identify and discuss various settings where OT is provided to the adult (20+ years).
- Use observation skills to gather objective data used in the assessment and evaluation of clients with developmental disabilities (children/adults).
- Participate in service-learning and collaboration with families, caregivers, and other professionals.
- Gather data for evaluation using assessment skills typical of practice by OTAs.
- Plan and implement therapeutic occupations.
- Analyze various activities/occupations and adapt and/or grade activities, accordingly.
- Develop and promote the use of home and community programming (accurate to individual need) to support performance in the individual's natural environment.

(continued)

Table 7-5 (*Continued*)

- Demonstrate entry-level competence in documentation skills typically exhibited by OTAs.
- Demonstrate accuracy in effective professional communication (verbal, nonverbal, written).
- Identify and access informational resources used in practice, including other healthcare provider roles.

processes of critical thinking and reflection to the surface for expression and discussion (Steele, 2007). Through this out loud reflection process, faculty can also model the type of reflection that we hope to facilitate in terms of critical thinking and questioning of assumptions regarding community and practice.

Table 7-6 illustrates examples of lessons learned and challenges in this course that provide opportunities for students, faculty, and community partners to come together to find creative, collaborative strategies, and solutions for the dynamic learning and growth that can occur through community engagement experiences.

Table 7-6 Challenges and Solutions.

Challenges	Solutions
Evaluation of student reflection can be subjective. The purpose of reflection evaluation is to see evidence that students are becoming more mindful, more thoughtful, and more appreciative of the conditions they see and the roles occupational therapy can play.	Group reflection has been beneficial to facilitating the reflective process and guiding critical-thinking and clinical-reasoning efforts.
Time demands continue to be an issue for students. They must initiate this process in a timely fashion and maintain a regular schedule in order to complete the service learning goals successfully.	Success is not achieved by simply getting the task done, rather it means that the learning process is engaged and the client or community partner is satisfied.

Interpersonal Skills for the Allied Health Professional

Service-learning is an integrated part of the Interpersonal Skills course. This is a one-credit class held in the spring semester. This course is a corequisite for Lifespan I. The service-learning activities are focused on professional interactions and marketing of occupational therapy and, in particular, the role of the occupational therapy assistant (Table 7-7).

Table 7-7 Occupation of Learning Through Service Engagement: The Syllabi.

COURSE NAME: Interpersonal Skills for the Practicing Allied Health Professional

COURSE DESCRIPTION: The purpose of this course is to increase awareness and develop understanding of interpersonal and intrapersonal skills as they relate to the Allied Health Professional. The focus is to enhance communication skills essential for positive and effective therapeutic and professional relationships in the healthcare field. Particular emphasis will be placed on self-awareness, therapeutic use of self, values clarification, verbal/nonverbal communication, written communication, conflict resolution and dispute resolution methods, professionalism, and performance evaluation.

Service-learning objectives which support course objectives:
- To apply professional skills
- To use effective communication techniques
- Demonstrate personal management skills when working in a group (i.e., time management, etc.)

Pertinent Course Objectives relative to service learning objectives:

Upon successful completion of the course, the Allied Health student should have acquired knowledge, attitude, and skill that will enable each student to:
- Recognize the importance of nonverbal language in the healthcare setting.
- Develop a repertoire of effective communication skills that are applicable to a variety of challenging interpersonal and organizational situations.
- Examine and compare the boundaries of personal and professional communication.
- Demonstrate an understanding of the importance of effective interpersonal skills in the professional world.
- Use principles of time management, including being able to schedule and prioritize workloads.

The purpose of the service-learning experiences in this course is to apply professional skills and effective communication techniques, in the context of a group marketing project for occupational therapy month. This is a community activity that requires total number of six hours of service. Learning to show versus discuss the value of occupational therapy is an important aspect of this service-learning component.

Students receive this assignment at the beginning of the spring semester. It does not need to be carried out until April. This assignment is designed for groups of three to four people. Each group will choose to celebrate and share their knowledge of occupational therapy in April. This can be at the college, a facility, at the legislature, etc. As with any service-learning project in the OTA program, an intent paper precedes project initiation. Each project must include professionally written and accurately cited information. Each project must include at least six hours of the group's time *doing* the project. Each project must be assessed by the group/facility receiving the benefit from the project. Also, each group member is responsible to assess the performance of each person in the group. Groups will present project findings on the last day of class. Reflection incorporated in this course includes individual and group analysis of relational issues and techniques learned and attempted in this service-learning experience based on course objectives.

The group project described in the Interpersonal Skills for the Allied Health Professional course is a results-oriented project, but the process is integrated. Students have an opportunity to implement in real time and critically assess the importance of effective communication and professional behaviors. They create working links to classroom information while providing their communities information about occupational therapy. This project supports discussion regarding work ethics, team work, and individual characteristics of being an effective occupational therapy citizen (Table 7-8).

Table 7-8 illustrates examples of lessons learned and challenges in this course that provide opportunities for students, faculty and community partners to come together to find creative, collaborative strategies and solutions for the dynamic learning and growth that can occur through community engagement experiences.

Table 7-8 Challenges and Solutions.

Challenges	Solutions
Time constraints and individual time management	Faculty/individual group discussion of the value of preparation; brainstorming options; individual reflections, with faculty feedback, assists students in developing strategies.
Member roles which are undefined cause group task to breakdown.	Faculty/Individual group discussion of the abilities, styles of members and the needed roles; individual reflections.
Communication "learnings" that are not incorporated may cause conflict among group members.	Class and small group discussions emphasize the necessity of effective communication in working groups.
Fear of group grade.	A system is developed for individual grading within the group; grade reflecting individual work.

General Issues with Student Engagement

Based on our OTA program outcomes, students benefit in service-learning. Not unlike problem-based learning (PBL), students are learning new knowledge and immediately applying their newfound knowledge and skills (Seruya, 2007). Self-confidence, academic curiosity, and self-directed learning are enhanced in students in the OTA program who participate in service-learning. They begin to perceive themselves as professionals, thinkers, and problem solvers. Students are highly invested in the projects that they choose. Although choosing a site can be the most difficult part of the service-learning, it is here that students begin to understand their communities, their personal communication strengths and limitations, and their comfort in articulating occupational therapy (OT) practices. They also learn the skills that they need to initiate their own contacts and to accept responsibility for their learning, thus developing methods for enhancing student learning outcomes. They make a commitment to being active learners.

On occasion, sites are developed by the OTA program due to liability issues with certain populations. For example, if the student needs more guidance, the population/individual of interest to student is possibly unsafe, and/or the capacity for student learning and community satisfaction is negligible, the instructor will provide the safety net so the experience will provide the intended outcome. Although the initial contacts are made, the student is still responsible for connecting, articulating, and then implementing the service.

Through service-learning, students begin to use the theoretical foundations of OT as they engage, participate, and adapt. In order to ensure the integrity of the service-learning process, feedback and evaluation are critical. These are two processes used to promote and monitor the individual learning experience.

Additionally, providing students with regular feedback, based on the structure of the learning activities, assists students in assessing the quality of their interactions. Feedback is also a critical part of teaching students how to develop their reflection skills (Troppe, 1995). Feedback also helps students link their reflection skills to critical-thinking skills and builds future clinical-reasoning capacity. Feedback is provided as guidance from the faculty instructor and typically involves provocative questions for thought and therefore must be timely.

Evaluation of the Student in Service-Learning Experiences

Based on service-learning research and literature, there is no universally accepted evaluation methodology for assessing student service-learning outcomes; however, there is agreement that evaluation is essential. Evaluation provides a structured, systematic method for feedback; it also provides an opportunity for student accountability. Troppe (1995) discusses four components for effective evaluation:

1. Well chosen, clearly articulated goals and objectives on the part of the instructor
2. A means for students to communicate their experiences to the instructor
3. A measurement technique (for reflection)
4. Opportunity for the student to improve through feedback (p. 13)

Student evaluation in our service-learning projects is consistent with rubrics set in place for each course within the program for participation, professionalism, and grading. The service-learning components of all three classes have the same foundational threads that guide evaluation of student learning. The worksheets for Lifespan I and II are essentially the same. This has been helpful for student success. Through this coordination of forms, students are able to anticipate, self-initiate, and link the service-learning rationale more effectively for all service-learning experiences.

The fundamental forms are the:

- Intent paper
- Confidentiality statement/signature
- Reflection papers (instrumental for student success)
- Before service-learning begins
- During service-learning engagement
- After service-learning is complete
- Documentation of events
- Service-learning "Therapeutic Use of Self" (TUS) reflection statement

OCCUPATION OF LEARNING THROUGH SERVICE ENGAGEMENT

Importance of Student Reflection in Engagement

A key part of the learning experience using service-learning pedagogy is students are challenged to participate in owning their learning experience through reflection and collaboration with faculty and community partners. Students are encouraged to be active, engaged participants in their learning (Zlotkowski, 1998). We have seen this expressed in the service-learning experience. Students begin to take responsibility for their clients, their communities, and for their own decision-making. Students are better prepared for fieldwork and for future reasoning. Examples of student reflections that evidence these aspects of service-learning participation are provided in Table 7-9.

As we, occupational therapy practitioners, discuss the importance of engagement and participation in our client's lives, we as educators must be aware of the value of participation and engagement in the

Table 7-9 Examples of Student Reflections.

Student Reflection:

Before the Service-Learning Project:

What impact do you think you will have on the people you will be working with or for?

"I don't believe I will have an impact other than to meet people and make contact."

During the Service-Learning Project:

What topics from your class are you seeing in your service-learning project?

"I have discovered that I tend to finish peoples sentences for them and I have been working on this; I learned that a couple of the residents might be just looking for acceptance through their repeated vocalizations that they want to go home."

After the Service-Learning Project:

"I think OT would be useful for the caregivers more than for the clients, but we would be very useful in cueing their routines to help them do for themselves."

Student Reflection:

Before the Service-Learning Project:

What do you think your service-learning site will be like?

"I think it will be busy and buzzing with conversation so I will have to really test my communication skills."

During the Service-Learning Project:

What topics from class are you seeing in your service-learning?

"One thing our class recently learned about was transference and counter-transference. I can see how incredibly easily a client or a therapist could fall into this trap. There are certain people that remind me of people I have known in my past. It takes a lot of conscious effort to keep their identities separate from the memories I have and the feeling attached to those memories; mostly topics about active listening and using therapeutic use of self qualities-being an effective listener involves being empathetic and learning to attune yourself to the other person's situation and perspective."

After the Service-Learning Project:

Was your understanding of the class work enhanced, magnified, or made easier as a result of your participation in this project?

"It was definitely enhanced. I think that you are able to learn better if you can make a personal connection to the information presented and after working with people with mental illness I could do this."

(*continued*)

Table 7-9 (*Continued*)

Student Reflection:

Before the Service-Learning Project:

What are the issues that your project or the service site addresses?

"A woman with bipolar illness."

During the Service-Learning Project:

What topics from your class are you seeing in your service-learning project?

"Isolation."

"I have seen an increase in the client's motivation. She seems to be more eager to start new things—there is a different presence about her."

After the Service-Learning Project:

What have you learned from successes or disappointments in your project?

"I learned that the most caring of families do not always understand what their loved ones need."

Was your understanding of the class work enhanced, magnified, or made easier as a result of your project?

"I'd say yes because I often found myself picturing how certain things were related to my project. Having a specific environment to relate things to make it easier, I think."

Student Team Reflection:

Before the Service-Learning Project:

What impact do you think you will have on the people you will be working with or for?

"We hope to help people realize that OT is a resource in a variety of areas."

During the Service-Learning Project:

What topics from your class are you seeing in your service-learning project?

"One topic that we saw was the value for 'Quality of Life-Being, Becoming, Belonging' This concept was very apparent at this site. Each person was respected for who they were, accepted and offered chances to fulfill hopes and goals important to them."

What are the most difficult and satisfying parts of your service?

"Initially, it was difficult to develop a rapport with the site supervisor. After better communication the focus and expectations of the project—this problem was resolved."

After the Service-Learning Project:

Was your understanding of the class work enhanced, magnified, or made easier as a result of your participation in this project?

(continued)

Table 7-9 (*Continued*)

"Class work was enhanced by this project and this team project was enhanced by class work. Having had the Interpersonal Skills class—also gave us the ability to develop boundaries between personal feelings and professional aspects."

Overall Student Reflection on Service Engagement Experiences:

"I am very pleased with the end result of this project. I am hoping that the client's family fulfills its commitments to be more involved in her needs and care."

"I feel privileged to have met so many promising and creative young people, and to have donated time to my local community. I learned a great deal in a very unique setting that demonstrates the need for occupational therapy with young people out of traditional settings."

"I am able to see his progress or how the rest of his life unfolds. I am satisfied in my choice to work with him on this project because we both benefitted; I have helped him be more prepared to move on in school and life."

"I had doubts about this project beforehand, but I feel that I have benefitted from being given the chance to use the skills I have obtained."

"I learned a lot about writing SOAP notes and the importance of documentation. The regular feedback was really valuable. I feel better prepared for level one fieldwork."

"This service-learning experience has opened our eyes to how much of an impact we (OT practitioners) can have on society. This also reiterates the OT can be used in many different arenas, such as day programs to residential facilities. This project has made us feel that our knowledge and skills do make a difference to others. By using our skills and exercising our knowledge in the community, they will only have a positive impact on the members of society."

education of our students. We can contribute to building the evidence base for occupational therapy in part by supporting the value of experience. Thomas and Javaherian write, "As educators, we have the responsibility to personally reflect on our role in supporting and achieving the centennial vision" (2008, p. 3). Service-learning is one way to fulfill this role by preparing responsible future practitioners who use reflection, along with evidence, to meet the needs of clients.

Importance of Faculty Reflection on Engagement

Throughout any educational process, instructors support critical thinking in many ways: critiquing, appraising, and assessing through review and comment are typical methods of engaging a student to grow as a scholar. The importance of faculty reflection on service-learning engagement is no doubt equally as critical to supporting the development of students' critical and clinical reasoning ability. Boyt Schell (2008) writes about the importance of reflection as it relates to best practice: "A commitment to reflective inquiry as an integral part of our practice may be the best hope for living up to our own commitment to helping people" (p. 21). She further honors the value and importance of reflection as she discusses the complexities of practice problems and a practitioner's core assumptions about his or her practice. An educator has a pertinent role in advancing a student's ability in developing reflection skills. As noted by Boyt Schell (2008), "Given that reflection is part of [occupational therapy] practice, one must also consider that quality of reflection may vary among practitioners" (p. 20). Students can learn to improve the quality of their reflection by examining the elements of thought and through

Table 7-10 Faculty Reflection on Service-Learning.

- The more students understand the value of service-learning, the better they can articulate the project to community partners.
- The clearer the expectations, the better the outcome.
- Facilities may confuse service-learning with level I, level II Fieldwork—so be clear, very clear.
- Some students are not prepared to direct their own learning without assistance.
- Fear induces hesitation and impacts success for some students.
- Some students needs more structure than others.
- Student reflection is critical and sometimes needs to be nurtured.
- Students are used to tracking "progress"; reflection is a new concept for many.
- Time constraints vary for students, faculty and facilities. Service-learning can be an above and beyond time commitment.
- Confidentiality and HIPAA regulations must be reviewed and understood prior to service-learning.
- Safety concerns must be addressed and clearly articulated.
- Simultaneous service-learning projects for multiple courses can hinder the intent.
- Occupational therapy faculty may need to be flexible and work in tandem with other faculty (e.g., same project, different focus, intent, reflection, feedback, and guidance).

faculty feedback that is deliberate and mindful. Table 7-10 highlights the significant understandings of faculty reflection when supporting student engagement.

CONCLUSIONS

The occupation of learning through service engagement is a powerful connector for students. The expressed outcomes of service-learning experiences at KVCC include:

1. Service-learning improves the understanding of the value of being a reflective practitioner and critical-thinking outcomes.
2. Professional maturation as a whole increases.
3. Teaching/learning principles naturally occur with opportunity (case method, PBL, and collaborative method of learning and service-learning).
4. Initiation of individual learning, through choice of placement/population interest improves motivation and engagement.
5. Comfort level in decision making improves outside of the classroom, with opportunity.
6. Learning flexibility improves with service-learning opportunities.
7. Improved understanding of the human condition regardless of need/disability status is evident; people are seen as people first.
8. Fear (of some populations/experiences) diminishes with familiarity.
9. Engagement with a variety of nontraditional occupational therapy clientele provides for employment options for the future (e.g., adults with developmental disabilities, homeless shelters, small businesses, wellness populations).
10. Students can relate more positively to the anticipations/expectations of fieldwork (Levels I and II) especially for those who do not/have not had healthcare experience.
11. The ability to relate more effectively improves with opportunity.
12. Student's ability to articulately define occupational therapy increases.

13. The larger "culture of helping" is better understood.
14. Faculty feedback is valuable in demonstrating therapeutic qualities of specificity, immediacy, respect, genuineness, etc.

The purpose of this chapter was to demonstrate the value of service-learning in occupational therapy assistant education. Ideas and techniques to develop service-learning through community engagement have been discussed and insights shared about the value of service-learning in developing fieldwork readiness, reflection, and reasoning. Our role as educators is to teach students to be imaginative and resourceful occupational therapy practitioners who will be able to problem solve and find solutions for the ever-developing challenges and opportunities they will face as twenty-first-century practitioners.

Within our OTA program, we have learned as educators through community partnerships and service-learning experiences that students improve their ability to sort through problems in real time, utilizing the skills of many experts in many varied groups from many different perspectives. They learn to bridge the gap of theory and practice, using reflection to examine their rationales. We, as educators, provide a valuable facilitative function for teaching social responsibility, citizenship, and the meaning of participation and engagement in occupation.

REFERENCES

Beck, A. J., & Barnes, K. J. (2007). Reciprocal service-learning: Texas border Head Start and master of occupational therapy students. *Occupational Therapy in Health Care: A Journal of Contemporary Practice, 21*(1–2), 7–23.

Boyt Schell, B. (2008). The importance of reflection. *OT Practice, 13*(14), 20–21.

Campus Compact. (2000). *Service learning: Using structured reflection to enhance learning from service.* Providence, RI: Brown University.

Fenzel, M., & Peyrot, M. (2005). Comparing college community participation and future service: Behaviors and attitudes. *Michigan Journal of Community Service Learning, 12,* 23–21.

Hinck, S. S., & Brandell, M. E. (2000). The relationship between institutional support and campus acceptance of academic service learning. *American Behavioral Scientist, 43*(5), 868–881.

Kolbe, C. (Ed.). (1996). *Piecing our future together: Service learning in college courses: A resource guide.* Bedford, MA: Middlesex Community College.

Kennebec Valley Community College. (2001). *Kennebec Valley Community College faculty service-learning handbook.* Waterville, ME: Author.

Kennebec Valley Community College. (2008). *Student handbook & planner.* Waterville, ME: Author.

Kennebec Valley Community College. (2009). *KVCC OTA Student Handbook.* Waterville, ME: Author.

McGreal, I. (Ed.). (1992). *Great thinkers of the Western world.* New York: Harper Collins.

Schkade, J. K. (1999). Student to practitioner: The adaptive transition. In P. Crist (Ed.), *Innovations in occupational therapy education* (pp. 147–156). Bethesda, MD: AOTA.

Seruya, F. (2007). Preparing entry-level occupational therapy students: An examination of current teaching practices. *Education Special Interest Section Quarterly, 17*(4), 1–4.

Steele, V. (2007). Shared reflection in service learning. In P. Horrigan (Ed.), *Extending our reach: Voices of service learning at Cornell* (pp. 78–83). Ithaca, NY: Cornell Public Service Center.

Strange, A. (2000). Service learning: Enhancing student learning outcomes in a college-level lecture course. *Michigan Journal of Community Service Learning, 7,* 5–13.

Thomas, H., & Javaherian, H. (2008). The Centennial Vision and the Education Special Interest Section. *Education Special Interest Section Quarterly, 18*(1), 2–4

Troppe, M. (Ed.). (1995). *Connecting cognition and action: Evaluation of student performance in service learning courses.* Denver CO: Campus Compact/ECS.

Zlotkowski, E. ((Ed.). (1998). *Successful service learning programs.* Bolton, MA: Anker Publishing.

Chapter 8

Translating Service-Learning Theory into Practice in Occupational Therapy Education

Karen Atler, MS, OTR/L

Preparing future practitioners to meet the increasing complexities of health care is a current and very real challenge. Our society's changing healthcare needs will require practitioners to engage in complex problem solving, addressing such issues as health disparities, creating new models to incorporate health and prevention, while also learning to work collaboratively with other health professionals and local communities (Healthy People 2010; Pew Health Professions Commission, 1998). Both the Pew Health Professions Commission and the U.S. Surgeon General support the use of community-based learning to meet this challenge. Service-learning, one form of experiential community-based education, provides an opportunity for students to assist with meeting community needs while simultaneously furthering their own learning and development (Jacoby, 1996). Despite the increasing use of service-learning in higher education (Campus Compact, 2000; Elmer, 2002), Abes and colleagues report that faculty do not attempt or continue use of service-learning in coursework because (1) they do not knowing how to implement it, (2) they have difficulty coordinating the experience, and/or (3) they lack the time to develop and implement service-learning (Abes, Jackson, & Jones, 2002). Being cognizant of these common deterrents, the author set out to create a realistic service-learning experience for a large number of students that could be maintained over time.

The two-year entry-level master's occupational therapy (OT) program at Colorado State University (CSU) is designed around the mission of the university, which is influenced by its land-grant heritage and is centered on a commitment to excellence in teaching, research, and service. Although service-learning is not a formal part of the OT curriculum, CSU has an active and supportive service-learning community.

Each year for the past five years, 40 to 60 students enrolled in Neurobehavioral Interventions II, a second-year occupational therapy course, have engaged in a service-learning project that is integrated into the course. This chapter describes the process of successfully designing, implementing, evaluating, and refining the service-learning project. Following a description of the course and the service-learning experience, the author will provide a look back at why and how the service-learning project was initially designed and how it has evolved. Service-learning principles and strategies that provided guidance during the development and evolution will be discussed. The next section describes the logistics of the current service-learning project, which includes identifying and matching participants from the community with students, managing ongoing communication, and integrating the experience with course content and structure. The chapter closes with the author's reflections on lessons learned and thoughts for future directions in using service-learning in occupational therapy education.

THE CONTEXT OF THE SERVICE-LEARNING PROJECT

At the time the service-learning experience was designed, the Neurobehavioral Interventions II course was one of six intervention courses in the OT curriculum focused on applying occupational therapy theory and practice to a specific population. Entry-level master's students take this course during their fourth and final semester on campus prior to starting their Level II fieldwork experiences. Most students have completed or are concurrently completing their third Level I fieldwork experience. During two of the three Level 1 fieldwork experiences, students spend time primarily observing and interacting with OT practitioners. The third Level I fieldwork experience combines community hours with a weekly faculty-led seminar. The community hours occur frequently at sites where occupational therapy currently is not being practiced or the role is changing or expanding.

As with all of the major intervention courses in the OT curriculum at CSU, the Neurobehavioral Intervention II course is a four-credit course. The three-hour lecture/recitation is held once a week with all enrolled students. In addition, students meet once a week for a two-hour lab in smaller groups (usually around 20 per section). The major course outcomes relate to students understanding the impact of neurological conditions on daily life and being able to apply the OT process in its entirety using sound clinical reasoning. Prior to the incorporation of service-learning into the course simulated cases were used in order to provide students an opportunity to apply occupational therapy assessments and intervention principles to adults who have experienced neurological conditions.

The Conception of the Service-Learning Project

Many of the common neurological conditions that impact adults, such as stroke, brain injury, multiple sclerosis, and Parkinson's disease are complex conditions that can impact multiple bodily systems (i.e., motor, sensory, and/or cognitive) and frequently have a long-term impact on the person and his or her ability to engage in daily life (Brown, Gordon, & Spielman, 2003; Clark, 1993; Elliott & Velde, 2005; Harris & Eng, 2004; Lundmark, 1996; Sabari, 2001). In addition, the common picture of how the condition impacts performance and participation in daily life varies tremendously, which makes it difficult for students, and even entry-level occupational therapy practitioners, to understand condition complexities. Previously enrolled students consistently gave suggestions/recommendations for integrating more "real examples" of people who had neurological conditions into class content. Students commented that it was difficult to grasp and understand the impact of these conditions and to "see" what the symptoms looked like in the absence of a real-world example.

As the instructor of the course, the author strongly believes in the core belief of our profession: that learning occurs through doing. In occupational therapy education, learning through doing, or active learning, is described as "a philosophical approach to teaching that facilitates deep, meaningful learning by engaging students in manipulating knowledge" (Griffiths & Ursick, 2003, p. 1). Active engagement and reflection have been identified as methods to enhance the thinking used by occupational therapists (Cohn & Czycholl, 1991; Griffiths & Ursick, 2003) and are also key elements of service-learning (Weigert, 1998). Recently, there has been an increase in allied health studies examining the impact of service-learning (active learning with reflection) on students' learning (Beling, 2003; Fruhauf, Jarrott, & Lambert-Shute, 2004; Gitlow & Flecky, 2005; Greene, 1997; Kramer et al., 2007; Mayne & Glascoff, 2002; Reising, Allen, & Hall, 2006; Scott, Harrison, Baker, & Willis, 2005; Weinreich, 2003; Wittman, Conner-Kerr, Templeton, & Velde, 1999; Younghee, Clasen, & Canfield, 2003). Each of these studies report positive changes in student outcomes, illustrating various ways of structuring learning and reflection, and reporting outcomes.

AN OVERVIEW OF THE SERVICE-LEARNING PROJECT

Being highly motivated to enhance the learning experience for students in the Neurobehavioral Intervention II course, the author applied for a Colorado State University Service-Learning Mini Grant.

Through this process, the author conceptualized the specifics of the project. The initial service-learning project was designed to allow students to spend time with an adult living with a neurological condition in order to support students' understanding of neurological conditions and occupational therapy's potential role. Identifying collaborating organizations (those in the community who could help locate adults living with a neurological condition who expressed a desire or need for services and were willing to participate) was an important first step. All community participants living with a neurological condition and not currently experiencing any acute health challenges who agreed to participate were included. If the community participant was not 21 years of age, the parents or guardian gave consent. The community participants' connections to occupational therapy services varied. Some had never received occupational therapy, whereas others were currently receiving outpatient or community-based occupational therapy services.

Once community participants were identified from a variety of community organizations/agencies, students were assigned in pairs. Although the specific activities students and community participants engage in has evolved over time, students have always been required to make multiple visits (four to six throughout the semester). After getting to know the community participant in the first few visits, students facilitated/supported the community participants' identification of and engagement in a chosen activity. Using a client-centered approach, the students got to know their community participant, individualized their approach, and allowed the community participant to be an active participant in setting goals and interventions (Harris & Eng, 2004; Law, Baptiste, & Mills, 1995; Stevens-Ratchford, 2005).

Table 8-1 provides an overview of the learning objectives, student activities, and assessment. The service-learning experience was integrated into the lecture portion of class by discussing problems and challenges, presenting stories, and showing video clips of occupational performance made from video captured by students with the participant's consent. Collaborating organizations (those who had assisted in locating community participants for the service-learning project) came to class to field questions as a way to provide closure.

Table 8-1 Initial Service-Learning Design.

Learning Objectives	Student Activities	Outcome Measures
Assess occupational performance.	Gather person's story. Observe performance.	Post stories on Web CT. Report performance.
Analyze occupation/ activity/task requirements.	Complete activity analysis.	Report activity analysis.
Plan, select, and perform intervention.	Help identify activity. Facilitate learning activity.	Project summary.

Although not specifically identified in the table, the majority of the assignments were added to already preexisting course requirements.

A MAJOR EVOLUTION

Adhering to one of the major guidelines of service-learning, that is, obtaining feedback from all constituents (Gelmon, Holland, Driscoll, Spring, & Kerrigan, 2001), students, community participants, and collaborating organizations were asked to provide feedback and recommendations on the service-learning experience. Formal student feedback was gathered using three methods: (1) a pre/post survey measuring change in perceptions of knowledge, skills, and confidence, (2) a post survey quantifying the benefits of the experience, and (3) open-ended questions allowing students to comment on benefits, challenges, and recommendations. Feedback from community participants was gathered by the students during their last visit. Using multiple-choice and open-ended questions, feedback related to the benefits and value of the project to both participants and students was gained. Gathering feedback from the collaborating organizations was the least structured aspect of this project. The project was informally discussed with each collaborating organization at the end of the semester either by phone or in person.

All constituents perceived the service-learning project very positively, but not without suggestions for change. Students identified the following as the greatest benefits of the service-learning component:

trying out aspects of the OT process, learning about conditions, and applying information learned in class. The greatest challenges were scheduling issues, working in "more difficult situations" (i.e., a person who could not communicate well, who was not very motivated, or who had cognitive deficits). The majority of students felt that the project should continue, but with modification. Recommended changes clustered around three major themes: (1) reordering classroom content to support student interactions in the community, (2) providing more supervision and connection with the instructor or staff from the collaborating organizations, and (3) examining logistics around time, scheduling, and number of assignments. Some of the staff from the collaborating organizations reported they were unclear as to their role with the students, but felt that the community participants benefited. Although the community participants were sometimes unclear as to what the project was about, the majority reported they would like to participate again.

Through examination of the feedback and taking time to engage in personal reflection, it became apparent to the author that the service-learning experience was missing a few important elements to provide a well-integrated service-learning experience for all constituents. Focusing first on the three unique characteristics of service-learning—reciprocity, balance, and reflection (Furco, 1996)—the author recognized that the original service-learning project was designed around the needs of the students in the classroom and had not started with an identified and stated community need, which is an important guideline in service-learning (Peterson, Yockey, Larsen, Twidwell, & Jorgensen, 2006; Romack, 2004).

Taking time to clearly identify the stated community need led to redesigning the activities that the students and community participants engaged in. Following important guidelines for best practice in service-learning (Witchger Hansen et al., 2007), the author took time to dialogue with several of the collaborating organizations who had referred people for the service-learning project. The author learned that some community participants needed additional assistance in order to participate in valued activities. Residents in a local assisted living community who had experienced a neurological condition were often not participating in valued activities due to residual dysfunction. Another organization providing supported employment for people with disabilities recognized that consumers often achieve greater vocational success if they engage in home and community activities. However, funding agencies do not pay for these types of services. If consumers could engage in home and community activities with support and encouragement from the students, the agency felt that not only would the consumers become more active, but in addition the agency would be better able to assess the consumer's work goal. Listening to these perspectives provided the instructor with greater clarity on how to create balance between service and learning.

At the time the project was redesigned, with the support of a second service-learning mini grant, the evaluation process expanded. Beginning with the identified need, the author examined and applied the "good practice" guidelines reported by Gray, Ondaatje and Zakaras (1999). Based on the results of the Learn and Serve America in Higher Education Program Evaluation (Gray et al., 1998), good practices guidelines were identified to provide guidance for developing effective service-learning experiences. The five guidelines are: (1) making a strong connection between course content and service, (2) volunteering more than 20 hours, (3) discussing the service experience in class, (4) providing training, and (5) providing supervision. The majority of these "good practices" guided the revisions.

Creating a seamless integration between the service-learning experience and course objectives and requirements was foremost. The author explicitly tied the service-learning activity to the course objectives and content, using the same language in both (see Table 8-2 and Appendix 8-A, Overview of Service-Learning). Reordering content supported students gaining background knowledge earlier in the semester. For example, many of the students worked with community participants who experienced cognitive challenges. The author rearranged the sequence of class content by providing an overview of motor, sensory, and cognitive-perceptual assessment and intervention focusing on adaptations within the first six weeks of the semester. A focus on remedial issues followed later in the semester. Streamlining and reducing the number of assignments and tying them directly to

Table 8-2 Overview of Major Revisions to Service-Learning Design.

Components of the Project	Original	Revised
Overview of key steps	Gather person's story. Observe perform-ance. Help identify activity. Facilitate learning activity.	Complete initial assessment: • Semi-structured interview • Observe performance • Collaborate to identify goal Implement plan. Reassess.
Assignments	Share story on Web CT. Report performance. Complete activity analysis. Write project summary.	Write assessment. Develop intervention plan. Write summary report. Report visits through e-mail. Write synthesis paper.
Integrating service-learning experience into class	*Lecture* Discuss stories, prob-lem areas, and progress. Show videos. *Closure* Field questions from community partners.	*Lecture* Integrate videos and discussion. *Lab* Discuss intervention plans. Discuss concepts applied to service-learning participants. *Closure* Discussion with peers and instructor.

course objectives continues to be a means of integrating service and learning (see Table 8-2). Although modifying assignments was a primary way to promote integration of service and learning, the instructor also created better opportunities in class for students to discuss and reflect upon their experiences while receiving feedback (Hatcher &

Bringle, 1997). Moving the discussion and reflection of the service-learning experience into the smaller lab sections instead of during lecture worked effectively and is still being used. Reflection of service-learning does not happen automatically, and needs to be explicitly designed to occur throughout the course (Hatcher & Bringle, 1997). This is particularly true in order to make service-learning discussions a natural part of the course rather than an add-on. The author will discuss this in more detail later in the chapter.

As stated earlier, the focus of the second service-learning mini grant was to expand the evaluation process used to assess the effectiveness and logistics of the service-learning project. Even though the author saw the positive impact on student learning after delivering the first service-learning experience (i.e., students were better able to describe the impact of neurological conditions on occupational performance and/or apply the OT process), the benefits to the community remained unclear. Using qualitative methods, the author interviewed 10 community participants following the second service-learning experience. A constant-comparative analysis revealed two themes related to the benefits of participating in the service-learning experience. The process of relating and actively engaging (theme 1) was just as important as the outcomes gleaned from the experience (theme 2). In the interviews, community participants described three types of outcomes: developing relationships, gaining insights about self and/or one's abilities, and tangible results (i.e., learning, being able to perform better). With the results of the evaluation, the author's committed to keep the project going because of its benefits to the community. Allowing and/or helping faculty to discover the benefits of service-learning is key to successfully institutionalizing service-learning (Hatcher & Bringle, 1997).

LOGISTICS OF CREATING A SEAMLESS INTEGRATION

In order to create a seamless integration between service and learning, two areas have required continual evaluation and modifications: (1) managing the project, and (2) integrating the project into the course. "Good practice" guidelines (Gray et al., 1999) again provided a context in which to assess the parameters put into place for managing the project and incorporating the project into the classroom.

Managing the Project

Minor changes have occurred each year to help streamline the administration of the project. There are several essential components to managing the project: locating community participants, matching students with community participants, tracking matches, and communicating clearly with all constituents involved. Approximately 25% of the community participants from each year's project agree to continue their participation. At the end of each project year, students obtain feedback from the community participants for recommendations and determine if they would like to be contacted again. If they express interest in continuing to participate, they are contacted about a month prior to the start of the next project. In addition, past collaborating organizations are contacted. Although several agencies/groups/ organizations have participated for three or four years, new relationships are continually being built. Expansion of sites has been in response to some expressing concerns about the increase in work and demands put on their staff by participating in the project. This issue is not uncommon and has been addressed in the literature by Long, Larsen, Hussey, & Travis (2001). They warn faculty to be aware of the "intrusions" and inconveniences that can occur with having students connected with community agencies. Clear, open, and consistent ongoing communication is essential.

Creating an infrastructure to support faculty in managing the logistics of service-learning has been identified as an important component of ensuring sustainability (Furco, 1996). During the first two years, graduate students were hired through the grant to assist the author in setting up the project (i.e., contacting participants, creating database files, filing, etc.). As the grant money ended, work-study students assisted with administrative tasks, and the author took on the primary role of contacting participants and managing the service-learning project. As the value and benefit of the project grew and was recognized within the OT department, support to recruit and assist with communicating with community participants, as well as track and manage the database, has been incorporated into the work load of a regular staff position. The author believes that several of the other factors presented by Furco (1996), in his discussion on factors that can influence the institutionalization of service-learning at the campus level, were influential in gaining departmental support for the service-learning project. These include ensuring that the service-learning is tied to the mission of the department and curriculum, and showing how service-learning has strengthened student learning outcomes.

Once potential community participants are identified and students have chosen a peer to work with and have expressed their preferences, students are matched with participants. Initial letters are now sent to community participants sharing the names of the students who will be contacting them. The administrative staff also sends students information about their community participant (written in a short biographical sketch) through e-mail. If community participants have been involved in the past, their previous goals and progress toward the goals are shared with the students. It is then up to the students to contact their participant and arrange the first meeting.

During the first meeting, the students re-explain the purpose of the project and have the community participant sign a consent form. In addition to confirming his/her agreement to participate, community participants also express what and how information can be shared. A portion of the consent form illustrating how the project is explained can be found in Appendix 8-A. The specific consent form is not shared, because most universities have specific guidelines or policies that must be followed.

To help students understand the service-learning project, a handout is provided during the first scheduled lab (see Appendix 8-B). The document states the purpose of the project, identifies the collaborating organizations, and describes what the students will be doing during each step of the project. A question-answer format posing frequently asked questions clarifies requirements, describes how to get started, offers resources available to support learning and service, and explains what to do if students are having difficulty during different phases of the project. Details regarding service-learning assignments, along with assignment formats and grading criteria, complete the handout. The last section provides an overview of the assignments, including assignment formats and grading criteria (not included in Appendix 8-B).

Following each visit with a community participant, the students e-mail the instructor and agency contact (if there is one). Students briefly summarize the focus of the visit (data), their impressions (interpretation), and what will happen next (plan). This provides the students with an opportunity for immediate reflection and practice with documentation, and the instructor is able to keep a "pulse" on what is happening and can intervene if needed. The instructor sends a brief e-mail back, immediately providing feedback or answers to questions. In addition, the instructor can track common issues or concerns that can be addressed during class with all the students. Although the author is unaware of others who have used this method of communication, Siefer and colleagues suggest using electronic discussion groups as a way to create opportunities for support, networking, and continuing education among faculty, collaborating organizations, and students (Seifer, Mutha, & Connors, 1995). The expediency of technology has assisted the author with managing the large number of students.

Integrating Service with Learning

Not only has the way the project is managed changed over time, the methods used to integrate the service-learning project into the course have evolved. Three methods are currently used: (1) assignments, (2) discussion in labs, and (3) videos. Three of the four lab assignments are related to the service-learning project, and one assignment is incorporated into the lecture course. In lab, the three assignments follow the OT process: evaluation, intervention plan, and summary (discharge) report. All lab assignments are completed collaboratively by the student pair, with each student receiving the same grade.

Tryssenaar (1995) states, "although reflection is individually centered, some authors have suggested that reflection in isolation is less effective than reflection in community through collegial interaction and dialogue" (p. 696). The majority of students report that working together outweighs the challenges.

The evaluation, summary reports, and final synthesis reflection are written assignments. Over the past five years, the instructor has changed the location and format of the synthesis reflection assignment; however, the final synthesis is done individually. Although a number of students state that they do not value the written reflection synthesis at the end of the semester, the author has found that oral reflection at the end of the semester is often hard to facilitate. For the most part, only a small portion of students in the class actively participate. Restructuring the written assignment has allowed the author to better assess students learning. Following guidelines to facilitate "reflection-on-action," the paper's requirements are clearly outlined (Eyler, Giles, & Schmiede, 1996; Silcox, 1993). Students briefly describe the service-learning experience and what they found challenging and rewarding. They then integrate their experience with five key concepts learned in class. After completing a self-assessment, students close by sharing what they will take from the experience as they begin Level II fieldwork.

Although the intervention plan was initially written, it is now presented orally, to simulate reporting during team rounds. Students are given five minutes to share their plan, followed by the instructor asking each student one question to promote and evaluate clinical reasoning. Change in the structure of the intervention plan assists in (1) balancing the amount of work required by students for a one-credit course, (2) streamlining the amount of time required for grading by the instructor, and (3) creating a way to promote sharing and discussion of all community participants.

In addition to taking time to discuss the intervention plans during lab, the author has identified other inherent ways to incorporate the service-learning experiences into lab and lecture. As discussed earlier, reflection does not occur automatically, but requires attention to ensure that it occurs throughout the course (Hatcher & Bringle,

1997). Plack and Santasier (2004) discuss the important role of reflection in learning, referring back to the work of Dewey (1938), Kolb (1984), and Schon (1983). According to Plack and Santasier (2004), "Many theorists concur with Dewey's concept that experience is the raw material for learning, adding the reflective process is what gives meaning to the experience" (p. 5). The author used the work of Dantonio (1990) to assist with using questions to integrate classroom content and service-learning experiences. For example, when content related to using everyday activity to assess motor control was presented, students were asked to share task observations made during the service-learning experience to illustrate how motor issues (strengths and challenges) influence occupational performance.

The most recent method used to promote discussion during lab was to have each student pair introduce their participant to the class after they completed their first visit. They shared how class content was used with the community participant. This set the stage for the remainder of the course. The expectation and hope was that students would share experiences throughout the course.

The third method for integrating service-learning experiences into classroom learning has been the use of video clips of community participants performing daily activities. After obtaining consent from community participants, some students videotaped either a portion of the assessment or the intervention provided. Videos were transferred to DVD and used during the course to help illustrate key concepts. In the nursing literature, video has been described as being useful in triggering discussion and assisting with skills training (McConville & Lane, 2006; Minardi & Ritter, 1999).

REFLECTIONS AND FUTURE DIRECTIONS

In writing this chapter, I have had the opportunity to reflect upon many aspects of the project. Amazingly, it has been five years since the inception of the project! Each year it evolves into a stronger, more easily managed project; however, it has not been without challenges along the way. Looking back, I can see and appreciate that developing a service-learning project takes time. My advice is to start small, establishing a simple project. Once it is developed, make only a few changes at a time. As Abes and his colleagues have summarized, people report that they do not continue using service-learning because of the challenges in coordinating the project. My hope is that you have learned from my process. I think that today's technology can help us manage the logistics of service-learning projects.

I could not have developed and refined such a successful project without accessing and using my available resources. Although you may not have many local or campus resources and supports, there are some great supports available on a national level. I would strongly encourage you to take the time for education and training. An unexpected reward for me has been finding a group of peers across various disciplines who are committed to promoting active learning through the use of service-learning. These peers can become great resources and supports.

Taking time to evaluate the project and seeking feedback from all constituents was essential to the development of the project. Remember to allow yourself time to reflect. As the instructor, your role and feedback is just as important as any other. It was not until writing this chapter that I reaffirmed the importance of starting with an identified and *stated* community need, not from one's limited perception of student needs (Bittle, Duggleby, & Ellison, 2002; Furco, 1996).

Although evaluation is an essential element of service-learning, I have not determined how to streamline the process to make it feasible, given the constraints of my other responsibilities and priorities. I feel that ongoing assessment is important, not only to guide changes made in the project, but also to demonstrate the effectiveness of service-learning as an educational method in occupational therapy. Eyler (2000) has stated that there is a need to define and measure the cognitive outcomes of service-learning, not just students' perceptions of the learning. In my brief evaluation, I focused on change in students' perceptions of their knowledge, skills, and confidence in working with clients with neurological conditions. In addition, Eyler has stated the need to explore how particular service-learning designs and techniques enhance the effects of service-learning. Although experimental designs are challenging, carrying out research projects across universities and learning communities may provide one way to use more rigorous designs to improve the research in this area.

Integrating the service-learning experience into the classroom has been the most challenging aspect of the project. There is a dynamic, ever changing balancing act between delivering content and supporting the process of learning. Another element that requires balance is deciding how much structure and support to provide while still allowing students the freedom to direct their own learning. I have found that if I provide strong structure and support, students are able to take on more challenges and direct their own learning. Without structured support, fear and insecurities impede learning. In summary, allowing students to direct their own learning does not eliminate the need for providing structure and support from an instructor's perspective.

I have also discovered that as an instructor I am more comfortable directing when and how content is covered, along with the need for a very clear and concise plan. However, in order to allow time for processing of the service-learning experience during class, I have learned you can't just keep adding content. When incorporating service-learning, I need to be willing to take some content out to allow room to integrate service-learning. In order to incorporate service-learning, it requires us, as instructors, to always be aware and willing to make connections to class content for the students, whether it is content we covered previously or content that still may be to come. All of these connections do take time. I appreciate Hooper's discussion on how education is often organized around a central focus, whether that is student-centered, expert-centered, or subject-centered (Hooper, 2006). For me, I need to remember to stay subject-centered—keeping occupation as my main method and focus of learning.

In summary, it has been amazing to watch the project grow and develop and gain increasing recognition within the department, both by students and administration. Please note the appendices at the end of this chapter for course syllabi and assignments. The interest in this project has led to discussions around other ways we might integrate community and fieldwork experiences within course content, thus meeting the new 2008 ACOTE standards requiring fieldwork to be an integral part of the curriculum. Although there has been a huge investment on my part, I feel that the service-learning project has enhanced students learning, helped meet a stated community need, and added to my enjoyment of teaching.

REFERENCES

Abes, E. S., Jackson, G., & Jones, S. R. (2002). Factors that motivate and deter faculty use of service-learning. *Michigan Journal of Community Service Learning, 9*(1), 5–17.

Beling, J. (2003). Effect of service-learning on knowledge about older people and faculty teaching evaluations in a physical therapy class. *Gerontology & Geriatrics Education, 24*(1), 31–46.

Bittle, M., Duggleby, W., & Ellison, P. (2002). Implementation of the essential elements of service learning in three nursing courses. *Journal of Nursing Education, 41,* 199–132.

Brown, M., Gordon, W. A., & Spielman, L. (2003). Participation in social and recreational activity in the community by individuals with traumatic brain injury. *Rehabilitation Psychology, 48*(4), 266–274.

Campus Compact. (2006). 2006 service statistics. Retrieved March 3, 2008, from http://www.compact.org/about/statistics/2006/service_Statistics. pdf.

Clark, F. (1993). Occupation embedded in a real life: Interweaving occupational science and occupational therapy. 1993 Eleanor Clark Slagle lecture. *American Journal of Occupational Therapy, 47*(12), 1067–1078.

Cohn, E. S., & Czycholl, C. (1991). Facilitating a foundation for clinical reasoning. In E. B. Crepeau & T. LaGarde (Eds.), *Self-paced instruction for clinical education and supervision: An instructional guide* (pp. 161–182). Rockville, MD: American Occupational Therapy Association.

Dantonio, M. (1990). *How can we create thinkers? Questioning strategies that work for teachers.* Bloomington, IN: National Educational Service.

Dewey, J. (1938). *Experience and education.* New York: Simon & Schuster.

Elliott, S., & Velde, B. P. (2005). Integration of occupation for individuals affected by Parkinson's disease. *Physical and Occupational Therapy in Geriatrics, 24,* 61–80.

Elmer, D. (2002). From river rambles to museum meanderings: Student motivation and service learning. Paper presented at the Annual Meeting of the National Communication Association, New Orleans, LA, November 21–24.

Eyler, J., Giles, D. E., & Schmiede, A. (1996). *A practitioner's guide to reflection in service-learning: Student voices and reflections.* Nashville, TN: Corporation for National Service.

Eyler, J. (2000). Studying the impact of service-learning on students. *Michigan Journal of Community Service Learning,* Special Issue, 11–18.

Fruhauf, C. A., Jarrott, S. E., & Lamert-Shute, J. (2004). Service-learners at dementia care programs: An intervention for improving contact, comfort, and attitudes *Gerontology & Geriatrics Education, 21*(1), 37–52.

Furco, A. (1996). Service-learning: A balanced approach to experiential education. In Corporation for National Service (Ed.), *Expanding Boundaries: Serving and Learning* (pp. 2–6). Columbia, MD: Cooperative Education Association.

Gelmon, S. B., Holland, B. A., Driscoll, A., Spring, A., & Kerrigan, S. (2001). *Assessing service learning and civic engagement: Principles and techniques.* Providence, RI: Campus Compact.

Gitlow, L., & Flecky, K. (2005). Integrating disability studies concepts into occupational therapy education using service learning. *American Journal of Occupational Therapy, 59*(5), 546–553.

Gray, M. J., Ondaatje, E. H., Fricker, R., Geschwind, S., Goldman, C. A., Kaganoff, T., et al. (1998). *Coupling Service and Learning in Higher Education: The Final Report of the Evaluation of the Learn and Serve America, Higher Education Program.* The RAND Corporation.

Gray, M. J., Ondaatje, E. H., & Zakaras, L. (1999). *Combining service and learning in higher education: Summary report.* Santa Monica: RAND Corporation.

Greene, D. (1997). The use of service learning in client environments to enhance ethical reasoning in students. *American Journal of Occupational Therapy, 51*(10), 844–852.

Griffiths, Y., & Ursick, K. (2003). Active learning and occupational therapy education. *OT Practice, 17,* 1–3.

Harris, J. E., & Eng, J. J. (2004). Goal priorities indentified through client-centered measurement in individuals with chronic stroke. *Physiotherapy Canada, 56*(3), 171–176.

Hatcher, J. & Bringle, R. (1997). Reflections: Bridging the gap between service and learning. *Journal of College Teaching, 45*(4), 153–158.

Healthy People 2010. (n.d.). Disability and secondary conditions. Retrieved June 10, 2006, from http://www.healthypeople.gov/publications.

Hooper, B. (2006). Beyond active learning: A case study of teaching practices in an occupation-centered curriculum. *American Journal of Occupational Therapy, 60*(5), 551–562.

Jacoby, B. (1996). Service-learning in today's higher education. In B. Jacoby (Ed.), *Service-learning in higher education: Concepts and practices* (pp. 3–25). San Francisco: Jossey-Bass.

Kolb, D. (1984). *Experiential learning: Experience as the source of learning and development.* Englewood Cliffs, NJ: Prentice-Hall.

Kramer, P., Ideishi, R. I., Kearney, P. J. C., Michelle E., Ames, J. O., Shea, G. B., et al. (2007). Achieving curricular themes through learner-centered teaching. *Occupational Therapy in Health Care, 21*(1/2), 185–198.

Law, M., Baptiste, S., & Mills, J. (1995). Client-centered practice: what does it mean and does it make a difference? *Canadian Journal of Occupational Therapy, 62*(5), 250–257.

Long, A. B., Larsen, P., Hussey, L., & Travis, S. S. (2001). Organizing, managing, and evaluating service-learning projects. *Educational Gerontology, 27*, 3–21.

Lundmark, P. (1996). Relationship between occupation and life satisfaction in people with multiple sclerosis. *Disability and rehabilitation, 18*(9), 449–453.

Mayne, L., & Glascoff, M. (2002). Service learning: Preparing a healthcare workforce for the next century. *Nurse Educator, 27*(4), 191–194.

McConville, S., & Lane, A. (2006). Using on-line video clips to enhance self-efficacy toward dealing with difficult situations among nursing students. *Nurse Education Today, 26*, 200–208.

Minardi, H., & Ritter, S. (1999). Recording skills practice on videotape can enhance learning—a comparative study between nurse lecturers and nursing students. *Journal of Advanced Nursing, 29*(6), 1318–1325.

Peterson, B. A., Yockey, J., Larsen, P., Twidwell, D., & Jorgensen, K. (2006). Service-learning projects: Meeting community needs. *Home Health Care Management & Practice, 18*, 315–322.

Pew Health Professions Commission. (1998). *Recreating health professional practice for a new century.* San Francisco: Pew Health Professions Commission.

Plack, M., & Santasier, A. (2004). Reflective practice: A model for facilitating critical thinking skills within an integrative case study classroom experience. *Journal of Physical Therapy Education, 18*(1), 4–12.

Reising, D. L., Allen, P. N., & Hall, S. G. (2006). Student and community outcomes in service-learning: Part 1—student perception. *Journal of Nursing Education, 45*(12), 512–515, 516–518.

Romack, J. L. (2004). Increasing physical activity in nursing home residents using student power, not dollars. *Educational Gerontology, 30*, 21–38.

Sabari, J. S. (2001). Quality of life after stroke: Developing meaningful life roles through occupational therapy. *Loss, Grief & Care, 9*(1/2), 155–169.

Schon, D. (1983). *The reflective practitioner: How professionals think in action.* New York: Basic Books.

Scott, S. B., Harrison, A. D., Baker, T., & Wills, J. D. (2005). Interdisciplinary community partnership for health professional students: A service-learning approach. *Journal of Allied Health, 34*(1), 31–35.

Siefer, S., Mutha, S. & Connors. K. (1995, Spring) Service-Learning in Health Professions Education: Barriers, Facilitators, and Strategies for Success. *Expanding Boundaries: Service-Learning,* 36–41.

Silcox, H. C. (1993). *A how to guide to reflection: Adding cognitive learning to community service programs.* Philadelphia: Brighton Press.

Stevens-Ratchford, R. G. (2005). Occupational engagement: Motivation for older adult participation. *Topics in Geriatric Rehabilitation, 21*(3), 171–181.

Tryssenaar, J. (1995). Interactive journals: An educational strategy to promote reflection. *American Journal of Occupational Therapy, 49,* 695–702.

Weigert, K. (1998). Academic service learning: Its meaning and relevance. In R. A. R. J. Howard (Ed.), *Academic service learning: A pedagogy of action and reflection.* (pp. 3–10). San Francisco: Jossey-Bass Publishers.

Weinreich, D. M. (2003). Service-learning at the edge of chaos. *Educational Gerontology, 29,* 181–195.

Witchger Hansen, A. M., Munoz, J., Crist, P., Gupta, J., Ideishi, R., Primeau, L., et al. (2007). Service learning: Meaningful, community-centered professional skill development for occupational therapy students. *Occupational Therapy in Health Care, 21*(1/2), 25–49.

Wittman, P. P., Conner-Kerr, T., Templeton, M. S., & Velde, B. (1999). The Tillery project: An experience in an interdisciplinary rural health care service setting. *Physical & Occupational Therapy in Geriatrics, 17*(1), 17–28.

Younghee, K., Clasen, C., & Canfield, A. (2003). Effectiveness of service learning and learning through service in dietetics education. *Journal of Allied Health, 32*(4), 275–278.

Sample Description of the Project Within a Consent Form

Enhancing Engagement in Life with a Neurological Condition
  Authorization for CSU Student Learning

I, _____, agree to spend time with students who are enrolled at Colorado State University, in the Department of Occupational Therapy (OT). The students are taking a course called Neurobehavioral Approaches II (OT 634/635). The purpose of our time together is twofold: For the student to learn from my experience living with a neurological condition, and for me to get support accomplishing something I want to do with increased autonomy.

I understand that one to two students will spend time with me over the next 8–12 weeks. They will visit at least 6 times and together we will decide on a time that is good for us to get together. During those visits, the students will interview me to learn about my life, how my illness/injury has impacted me, and what I have learned in the process. In addition to talking with me, I understand that the students will observe me doing activities and will also complete an assessment of my living environment (home assessment).

After getting to know me, the students and I will decide on one small goal to work toward. The students will then provide support to me as I attempt to reach the goal I selected. At the end of the project, I understand that the students will be asking me to give some evaluative feedback about the process regarding what I gained from participating in the project.

I understand that the students are interacting and observing for the benefit of learning, and will not take a primary role in making decisions related to my care. However, at my request, the OT students will provide me feedback regarding the information they have gathered, which may include recommendations and suggestions.

Overview of the Service-Learning Project

Enhancing Engagement in Life with a Neurological Condition
  A Service-Learning Project Associated with OT 634/635
  Purpose: The semester-long project provides students (in groups of two) an opportunity to get to know a person whose life has been affected by a neurological condition and support them working towards an identified goal. Completion of this project will assist students in meeting the following course objectives:

- Gather, interpret, and report assessment information
- Plan, implement, and report OT services
- Incorporate knowledge of neurological conditions and personal perspective
- Articulate sound rationale

COMMUNITY PARTNERS

The students will work with adults who have experienced a neurological condition and are associated with various community agency community partners. This collaborative effort, with several local community members, makes this project possible.

OVERVIEW OF THE PROJECT

Throughout the entire process (1) you are ALWAYS collaborating with your community participant and agency and (2) written work will be shared with the affiliating agency in most cases. The project involves spending a minimum of six visits over the course of the semester. Students are to report each visit by e-mail.

1. Students will complete an initial assessment: (a) administer the Canadian Occupational Performance Measure (COPM), (b) assess occupational performance through observation of two different activities, and (c) identify impacting factors. Interpret information and identify one realistic goal to be addressed.

   Examples of goals addressed in the past are:

   - Cooking two meals a week using energy conservation. (This person experienced MS and could no longer work and wanted to be able to help his spouse with meal. Fatigue interfered with his performance.)
   - Crocheting using adaptive methods/equipment. (This person experienced a stroke and only had the use of one hand.)
   - Write, respond, and send e-mail. (This person experienced memory and problem solving issues due to a brain injury.)

2. Present your intervention plan orally in lab.
3. After approval, implement the plan—include at least three separate visits.
4. Reassess performance and write a summary report.

DETAILS RELATED TO GETTING STARTED

- Student pairs will be assigned a participant.
- Contact and schedule a time to meet your participant.
- Re-explain the project and have participant sign consent form (see attached example). Make sure that you have them clearly share their preferences.
- Return consent form to instructor ASAP.

DETAILS RELATED TO SPENDING TIME WITH COMMUNITY PARTICIPANTS

- You will spend a minimum of six visits during the semester.
- Spend *at least the first two visits* getting to know the person and completing the initial assessment (interview, COPM, and observing occupational performance and factors that support or hinder). If the person agrees to be videotaped, turn in the tape ASAP.

Once you and your participant have decided on a goal and your plan is approved:

- Spend the *next three to four visits* helping the person reach the identified goal.
- On your *last visit* complete your reassessment and provide clear closure.

COMMONLY ASKED QUESTIONS AND ANSWERS

Do I really need to make six visits over time? Yes. The project is designed to allow you to get to know a person over time and hopefully help the person be able to meet a small goal leading to greater performance or satisfaction in an area of life. Each group will determine what works best for all participants to meet the stated outcomes.

How long does each visit need to be? There is not a required length of time. Each group will determine what works best for all participants to meet the stated outcomes.

What if my participant does not seem to understand the project? Each person has had the project explained to them and has agreed to participate. However, because some people with neurological conditions can have difficulty remembering and understanding concepts, you will need to clearly identify who you are and explain the project. If your participant has cognitive issues, keep communication clear and simple. Each visit, share who you are, the purpose of project, and what you are going to do that day. As you end the visit, summarize what has happened, when you will meet next, and what you will do.

Ask the person how they learn best and use this method during your interactions (i.e., writing things on a calendar, leaving a note, calling to be reminded).

What if my participant does not want to be videotaped? Turning in a videotape of the participant's performance is NOT required. Refer back to the consent form if you or the participant has questions. The purpose of videotaping is to bring back some of your experience into the classroom for others to learn from.

Can I use the department's video equipment? YES. If you have signed a release, you may check out equipment **for a 24 hour period** of time. RESERVE USE AHEAD OF TIME to guarantee a camera. If you check out equipment over a weekend, you may need to coordinate with other students to share the resources. If you do not know how to use the equipment, resources for training are available. Please get training prior to videotaping.

Can I use the resources here in the OT department? YES.

- Most of the equipment in the closet downstairs can be checked out for a 24 hour period. Follow the procedures found in the student handbook.
- The technology in the ATRC may be used. Notify ATRC AHEAD of time as to when you will be bringing the person in, as well as what resources you will want to access. PLEASE NOTE that staff will not be available to help you learn the technology or problem solve.
- The OT garden may be used. Please reserve use of the garden space with your instructor. For use of gardening equipment follow the procedures for general supplies in the closet as stated above. Contact your instructor for specific garden tasks to work on.

What if I have concerns about my participant or am having trouble helping my participant identify a goal? Contact your agency person identified AND/OR the instructor. Leave an e-mail and phone message for them with a way to contact you. Clearly state the concerns and/or challenges and what you have attempted thus far. Make sure to share your rationale behind what you have done.

What if I have general questions about the project or assignments? ASK THE INSTRUCTOR. Either e-mail questions, set up an appointment, or ask questions during class.

DETAILS RELATED TO REQUIRED ASSIGNMENTS

Report Each Visit

Following EACH VISIT, take five minutes to e-mail a SHORT SUMMARY to the instructor AND agency contact person (if there is an agency contact, e-mail and phone number will be provided). **DUE: within 24 hours of each visit.** Use an informal format for a progress note: Data (What you and your participant did), Interpretation (your assessment of the time—focus on participant's performance), and Plan (what you will do next time). This is YOUR opportunity to work on writing brief but informative progress notes. They will not be graded. It will be OUR main opportunity to supervise and guide you. If you NEED more guidance or have questions, ASK.

Initial Assessment (done as a pair)

Write up your initial findings using the Assessment Form (see attached forms). You will gather the information to include on the assessment form during the first few visits you make with your participant. The primary methods you will use are: (1) informal interview, (2) completion of the COPM, and (3) observation of performance. Type the report. Do not exceed three pages double-spaced.

Oral Intervention Plan (done in pairs)

Prepare and share your intervention plan orally. Use the Intervention Form to assist you in planning your presentation (see attached forms). You will be given **five minutes** to share your plan. Think of this as if you are reporting during team rounds. Briefly share: (1) the occupational challenge and impacting factor, (2) the goal, (3) the strategies for working towards your goal, and (4) the rationale (why are you doing what you are doing and what do you expect to happen.

Make sure you connect your discussion to the factors you identified in the assessment that are leading to the occupational challenges). When you list your strategies you will support them using evidence from the literature. You each will then answer one question posed by the instructor to clarify or expand your report. Provide at least two evidence-based references (beyond resources used in class) to support your ideas. *Students will sign up for a time in lab during weeks 6–8.*

Summary Report

Write a summary using the Summary Form (see attached forms). Include the following: number of visits, baseline status, what was done, ending status, recommendations. Type the summary. Do not exceed three pages, double-spaced.

Reflection Synthesis OT 634

Reflection Synthesis (20% of total lecture grade)

Write an essay addressing the areas identified below. Your reflective discussion needs to address both your personal service-learning (s-l) experience as well as course concepts/principles. The expectation is that you will integrate your service-learning experience with readings and classroom learning. Evaluation criteria are identified below.

Paper length: 4–6 pages. Paper is to be typed and double-spaced.

Describe your service learning experience: Share your experience as if you were talking to a friend.

A. Briefly describe the context of your learning (who you worked with, what you did – do not repeat your summary report but summarize your experience in a paragraph).

B. Describe what you found most challenging and rewarding.

Integrate your service learning experience with course content:

A. Describe and apply five concepts/principles discussed in class or in your readings to your service learning experience. Concepts may be related to the impact a neurological condition on daily living, or any aspect of the OT process (e.g., observing, planning, documenting, and professional reasoning). Be sure to:

- Define the concepts in your own words and
- Apply the concepts to your service-learning experience:

  i. Describe how you saw the concept in action and
  ii. How you used class content during your s-l experience.
B. Compare and contrast classroom/reading content with your service-learning experience:
  i. In what ways was content and s-l experience similar? Different?
  ii. What are the possible reasons for the differences?

Evaluate your personal experience and learning:

A. Describe what you learned about:
  i. The people (and condition) with whom you worked. Do you feel differently about them now than you did when you started the project?
  ii. Engaging in the OT process
  iii. Our community
  iv. Yourself, your own strengths and limitations

B. What will you take from this experience as you begin Level II fieldworks?

Share your thoughts for future service learning experiences:

A. How would you change the service-learning experience to make it a more valuable learning experience?
B. What suggestions do you have for me and how I can be more effective in facilitating your learning from this experience?
C. What suggestions do you have for us as a program as we look forward to integrating more active learning into the curriculum?

Requirements	Evaluation Criteria
• Four to six pages • Typed and double-spaced • Organized and well developed	• **Completeness:** Did I answer all the questions? • **Accuracy:** Is my information factually correct and do I support with evidence? (This is related to course content.) Do I reflect evidence of meeting the course objectives? • **Clarity:** Do I expand on ideas, provide definitions and examples? • **Depth:** Do I explain my thinking and conclusions? Do I anticipate the answers to questions that my reasoning might raise? Do I acknowledge the complexity of issues?

Chapter 9

Occupational Therapy Service-Learning and Early Childhood Education

Roger I. Ideishi, JD, OT/L

This chapter describes a year-long service-learning partnership between an entry-level master's degree occupational therapy education program and an early childhood education center. This year-long service-learning experience involves integration among a curricular framework, two occupational therapy courses, and a community partner. The two-course integration involves creating continuity between two different, yet related, topical courses. The community integration involves a partnership that blends theory, practice, and education. The integration of curricular, course, and community components contributes to rich professional development opportunities for occupational therapy faculty, practitioners, and students.

The service-learning experience occurs at an inclusive Head Start preschool and is embedded in the laboratory sections of two courses:

Human Development and Performance in the fall semester and Human Occupation—Concepts and Practice in the spring semester. Ecological models of development and performance guide the service-learning experience in these two courses (Bronfenbrenner, 1999; Dunn, Brown, & Youngstrom, 2003). An assumption of this service-learning experience is that occupational therapy (OT) students understand how people participate in society through their own engagement in and perception of the world. If a student's perception of the self or environment is narrow, then a student's repertoire of response will also be narrow. Whereas, if a student's perception is broad then the student's repertoire of response will also be broad. A broad perception of the self or environment assumes the student has the opportunity and ability to engage in a diversity of environments (see Figure 9-1). Increasing a student's repertoire or environmental opportunities are goals of an ecological approach (Bronfenbrenner, 1995, 1999; Dunn, Brown, & Youngstrom, 2003). Using the concepts of an ecological model, the learning activities are designed to facilitate complex interactions between the student and the physical and social environment. These interactions inherently increase in complexity over time, occur weekly for the entire academic year, and invite attention, exploration, manipulation, elaboration, and imagination (Bronfenbrenner, 1999).

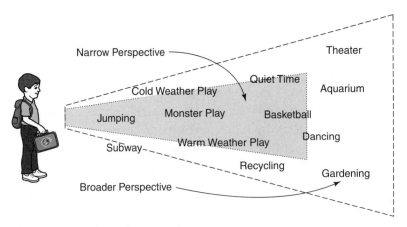

Figure 9-1 Ecological Perspective.

The service-learning opportunities broaden a student's perception for increasing the repertoire of actions. Because many students enter the field of occupational therapy with little to no professional clinical experience, this approach offers a flexible educational environment with meaningful experiences for a student to explore and expand her or his professional repertoire. Before participating in a clinically oriented fieldwork experiences, this service-learning experience provides the student the opportunity to develop and focus on self-reflection and interpersonal communication skills as a primary objective of the experience. Self-reflection and interpersonal communication are the foundation for building a year-long service-learning experience.

COMMUNITY PARTNERSHIP

This service-learning experience is the result of a partnership between KenCrest, a community-based service provider for people of all ages with developmental disabilities, and the entry-level master's occupational therapy program at University of the Sciences in Philadelphia (USP). KenCrest's Children and Family Services division serves infants, toddlers, and preschoolers who have developmental, neurological, orthopedic, behavioral, and learning difficulties in an inclusive setting at Head Start and Early Intervention centers. The missions of both institutions include serving the needs of the community. This mutuality forms the foundation for quality, early childhood education and the practice and education of occupational therapists. Community partnerships involve a shared commitment toward a mutual objective (Witchger Hansen et al., 2007). In this case, the objective was to create rich preschool learning opportunities and environments for children to explore, manipulate, elaborate, and imagine (Bronfenbrenner, 1999). This partnership has resulted in designing and building learning gardens, manufacturing playground equipment, creating community outdoor mosaic art, and developing a cultural arts program. For more information on these projects, see Ideishi, Ideishi, Gandhi, and Yuen (2006); Kramer et al. (2007); and Lorenzo-Lasa, Ideishi, and Ideishi (2007).

The Head Start preschool uses the High Scope curricular model to plan, evaluate, and guide children's learning. The High Scope model emphasizes active learning, independent thinking, and creativity in a rich environment structured with daily routines. The High Scope model believes learning is a social experience that encourages child-initiated learning through opportunity and choice. Shared child–adult control of the learning experiences is a quality of this model. This shared control promotes child-initiated exploration and creativity (Hohmann & Weikart, 2002).

USP OCCUPATIONAL THERAPY CURRICULUM

The USP OT program integrates service-learning throughout the curriculum. Service-learning experiences are required components for five courses, as well as additional service-learning opportunities in elective courses. The USP OT student spends up to 144 hours engaged in service-learning during the first professional year. A curriculum of this type requires a structure and schedule allowing for the extensive infusion of service-learning. The USP OT curricular themes provide the structure for developing service-learning. The USP OT curricular themes are clinical reasoning, critical thinking, innovations in practice, and engagement (University of the Sciences in Philadelphia, 2008). Service-learning experiences contribute, in part, to the foundation for these themes. Service-learning promotes critical thinking through deep reflection of the social, cultural, political, and economic contexts of occupational therapy practice. Service-learning promotes innovations through challenging future OTs to create or expand rich occupational therapy practices. Service-learning promotes engagement through regular participation in civic, health, and educational needs of a community (Kramer et al., 2007). These service-learning values are incorporated into the program's curricular objectives (see Table 9-1).

Service-learning is time intensive. The USP OT schedule provides weekly three-hour laboratory sections for the courses with service-learning. A program director's leadership and faculty investment to creative scheduling contributes to creating extended time blocks in

Table 9-1 USP OT Curricular Objectives That Support Service-Learning.

1. Successfully work in partnership with individuals from diverse populations.
2. Collaborate skillfully with clients, professionals, families, and community members.
3. Demonstrate an ability to be a reflective individual.
4. Provide service to the community.

the scheduling process. The curricular themes of critical thinking, innovations, and engagement were the driving force behind the faculty's development of a professional curriculum embedded with service-based experiences. The USP program director and faculty believe quality education and pedagogy drives curricular development. Creative problem solving balances administrative constraints with faculty teaching and learning philosophies. Three-hour learning labs are scheduled for each of the service-based courses. These labs and lab scheduling provide the flexibility to design service experiences with community partners. If service-learning is embedded as an effective pedagogy to address the curricular themes, faculty commitment can be naturally harnessed.

SERVICE-LEARNING COURSES

During the first professional year, two courses are involved in the Head Start preschool service-learning experience. The first course is Human Development and Performance during the fall semester. The second course is Human Occupation—Concepts and Practice during the spring semester. These two courses are sequential, but the Human Occupation course is not a continuation of the Human Development course. Both courses have a weekly three-hour in-class didactic active-learning lecture and three-hour service-learning lab at the Head Start preschool. Between the two courses, the OT student spends 72 hours engaged in service-learning at the Head Start preschool from September to April.

Human Development and Performance

The Human Development and Performance course is designed to provide an overview of the physical, cognitive, emotional, and sociocultural aspects of human development with an introduction to the analysis of developmental changes during human occupational performance of play, work, and self-care activities. A logical consistency of the course objectives, learning activities, and assessments is critical for integrating the service and learning expectations (see Table 9-2). The service-learning activities include writing four to five reflection papers, designing and leading preschool group activities, preparing a preschool child developmental analysis report, and planning a service project based on the community needs. The group activities and project have to be consistent with the preschool High Scope curricular model. Therefore, the students and preschool staff work collaboratively to ensure this match.

Table 9-2 Sample Human Development and Performance Objective–Activity–Assessment Integration (Fall Semester).

Course Objectives	Service-Learning Activity	Assessment Activity
Describe the acquisition, change, and adaptation of functional skills and abilities.	Collaborate with preschool teachers to propose, design, and implement five to six classroom activities.	• Activity proposal plan • Developmental analysis report • Five reflection papers • Preschool staff feedback survey
Describe the development and adaptation of self-care, play, vocational/productive abilities, and the influence of culture and society on these functional abilities.	Collaborate with preschool teachers to propose a community project for the preschool.	• Project proposal plan • Monthly progress and reflection note • Preschool staff feedback survey

The service benefit for the preschool is the additional assistance of human resources for classroom management, designing novel preschool activities, and addressing unmet community needs. The learning benefit for the OT students is the opportunity to apply and analyze their knowledge of human development and performance in a natural context and develop deeper reflective abilities.

Human Occupation—Concepts and Practice

The Human Occupation course is designed to explore the meaning and purpose of human occupation. The course examines and analyzes activities, habits, roles, and occupations for individuals with varying abilities. The laboratory emphasizes engagement in occupations within various social and cultural contexts. Similar to the Human Development course, a logical consistency exists between the course objectives, learning activities, and assessments (see Table 9-3). The service-learning activities are similar to the Human Development course.

Table 9-3 Sample Human Occupation and Performance Objective–Activity–Assessment Integration (Spring Semester).

Course Objective	Service-Learning Activity	Assessment Activity
Analyze activities and occupations in relation to areas of occupation, performance skills, performance patterns, and contexts.	Collaborate with preschool teachers to propose, design, and implement weekly classroom activities (12 weeks).	• Activity analysis report • Case report • Monthly reflection paper • Preschool staff feedback survey
Explain the impact of performance skills and performance patterns for engagement in occupations to support activity and social participation in context.	Collaborate with preschool teachers to design and implement community project for the preschool.	• Monthly progress and reflection note • Project analysis reflection paper • Preschool staff feedback survey

These include writing three reflection papers, designing and leading preschool group activities, preparing a preschool child case report, and implementing a service project based on the community needs. The student's familiarity with the assignment expectations and format from the previous semester provide a foundation to increase the student's complexity and depth of interactions with the community partner. As indicated in Table 9-3, the learning assignments are similar, but the learning assessments have a different focus. The spring semester goals are to continue building the relationship rather than restarting with new types of student-learning assignments. The focus of the spring semester assignments are the contextual influences on human occupation. In the previous semester, the students analyzed activities and occupations from specific components of human development and kinesiology.

PROCESS AND OUTCOMES

The results of this six-year Head Start–University partnership were the student activities and projects integrated into the preschool curriculum. These include gardening, dance education, and arts organization and museum partnerships.

The gardening program emerged from the staff expressing a desire to improve the aesthetics and safety of the preschool outdoor area. The former outdoor area was often strewn with pet waste, broken glass, syringe needles, and condoms. The OT students consulted with the preschool staff and then designed and built garden boxes, a sitting arbor, picnic tables, and a butterfly garden habitat in the outdoor space. The OT students implemented garden-themed indoor and outdoor activities that were integrated into the weekly lesson plans. The garden design and activities emerged from a theoretical analysis of the ecological interactions among various elements in, surrounding, and impacting the preschool (Dunn, Brown, & Youngstrom, 2003). Funding and resources were obtained through local community donations from lumber yards and home and gardening stores. Students searched for, wrote, and received small grants from regional philanthropic organizations to support these efforts.

The dance education program emerged from students using their background and interest in ballet and folk dancing to design class activities. Weekly dance classes were scheduled into the classes' gross motor play time. These dance activities were often matched to animal themes to motivate the children to experiment with new movement. Lorenzo-Lasa, Ideishi, & Ideishi (2007) report case examples from these dance experiences of children with autism and attention deficit disorder responding to the dance class with increased participation, attention, imagination, and social interaction. The OT staff continued the weekly dance program through grants from local foundations.

These curricular enhancements also initiated arts organization and museum partnerships. The preschool partnerships include attending the regional ballet company's dress rehearsal performances, the regional aquarium designing educational kits for children with autism and their families with the preschool staff and OT students, a regional theater bringing abbreviated stage performances to the preschool, and the preschool children participating in museum art workshops.

The preschool staff has added to the children's repertoire of opportunities through the collaboration and efforts with the OT students. In return, the OT students gained valuable experience in collaborating with community partners, writing small foundation grants, understanding children's activities and occupations, and understanding how to ground reasoning in a theoretical analysis.

CHALLENGES

Witchger Hansen et al. (2007) identified various challenges in creating service-learning experiences, such as interpersonal relationships between students and community members and establishing and reestablishing the relationship with each new student group. These were the same challenges for this Head Start service-learning program.

The OT students have to blend into existing preschool performance patterns. These performance patterns are sometimes explicit, such as the daily or weekly schedule of classroom activities. Many times these performance patterns are implicit, such as preschool staff speaking to children and other staff in non-English languages, how to manage a classroom, how to console a crying child, or how messy a child is allowed to get while painting. These implicit performance patterns have cultural influences that the OT student was often not aware of. Student and preschool staff orientation was an effective means to bridging these transitional issues as well as way of facilitating dialogue about common goals and expectations.

Another strategy to assist the OT student in this transition was to discuss the student's role in service-learning. For this Head Start experience, the student role was characterized as a teacher's helper. The OT student and course instructor dialogued about what it means to be a teacher's helper and what specific behavioral actions are associated with a teacher's helper. Topics related to culture, personal values and judgments, and physical touch are typically discussed. Other less complex roles and actions such as personal hygiene, cleaning the tables, or sweeping the floors are also discussed.

Prior to the start of the new academic year, the course instructor meets with the preschool staff to communicate each other's objectives and establish mutual objectives (Suarez-Balcazar, Muñoz, & Fisher, 2006). These meetings often produce the seeds for the students' community projects.

Initially, the course instructor serves as a liaison between the student and the preschool staff, helping to establish schedules or to coordinate a student-designed activity with the preschool teacher. This initial intermediary role-modeling allows the student to observe communication between the course instructor and preschool teacher. In time, the student assumes a more active and self-initiated role in the communication with the teacher. This process also allows the student and the course instructor to individualize the student's plan of action for establishing or deepening the student–teacher relationship. The course instructor's role also serves as the consistent element at the preschool to help both students and teachers bridge the transition of new students at the start of each academic year.

SERVICE-LEARNING COMMUNITY AND STUDENT ASSESSMENT

The assessment activities for the Head Start service-learning experience are listed in Tables 9-2 and 9-3. Formative assessments focus on the learning process whereas summative assessments focus on specific achievement or outcomes (Witchger Hansen et al., 2007). The formative assessments are the reflective notes or papers. The summative assessments are the proposal plans, progress notes, analysis and case reports, and preschool staff surveys.

The formative reflective assessments were chosen because of the student's year-long exposure to the service experience. The longer exposure allows for thoughts to be challenged and to change over time; therefore, the assessment should reflect this process (Witchger Hansen et al., 2007). Guided reflection was specifically used for the formative assessments (Ash & Clayton, 2004). Guided reflections were weekly instructor-generated questions rather than open-ended reflective thoughts (see Table 9-4). Kesler-Gilbert (2003) defines

Table 9-4 Sample of Instructor-Generated Guided Reflection Questions.

1. Describe a significant event from the day.
2. What elements from this week's course material did you observe or think about while interacting with the children at the preschool?
3. Were you relating and organizing the significant event to an occupation-based theoretical perspective? If so, which theoretical perspective do you tend to frame your observations?
4. How comfortable did you feel with your interactions and communication with the children and teacher?
5. What is your plan to increase your comfort or deepen your relationship with the children and teacher?
6. What are your impressions of educational inclusion?

guided reflections as an interactive communication that is connected, continuous, challenging, coached, and contextualized. Guided reflection helps the student to address and focus on the issues relevant to the course learning objectives (Ash & Clayton, 2004).

The summative assessments were chosen to measure the degree that student's achieved specific target actions and course objectives, such as developing the skill of activity analysis, planning an activity, observing actions and behaviors, and organizing observations into a comprehensive report. It is important to ensure cohesion between the course objective, learning activity, and assessment process. A grading rubric was developed based on the learning activity objectives.

Preschool staff surveys were distributed at the end of each academic year (see Table 9-5). The preschool staff's completion of the assessment survey and their contributions to designing the student experience are indicators that a stable and mutually beneficial relationship exists between the university and the preschool (Bringle & Hatcher, 1996). Based on the annual survey results, the course instructor, preschool director, staff occupational therapist, and preschool teachers adapt and modify the next experience to improve the experience for both the student and staff.

Table 9-5 Community Rating Survey Statements.

Rating Scale: Strongly Agree, Agree, Not Sure, Disagree, Strongly Disagree

1. It was difficult coordinating the efforts of the staff and students for the service-learning experience.
2. Orientation to the community experience is an important component of service-learning. Students were well oriented to my agency and client population.
3. Students were effective in the work they did for my agency.
4. In comparison to the usual volunteers, I had to spend more time and effort devoted to this experience.
5. The time spent with the students was worthwhile/valuable/time well spent.
6. If given the opportunity, I would choose to do a service-learning experience with a student again.

Please provide additional comments.

An example of a modification as a result of the community survey included the addition of the Developmental Analysis and Case Report. Prior to the addition of these assignments, the students only completed regular reflection papers. Unbeknownst to the OT student, the fall reflection papers typically addressed a continual narrative of the student's observations and experience with the same child. Students often had difficulty linking their reflection papers into a continuous story about the child. Preschool staff reported positive, yet moderate, effort in guiding students to link their class observations. As a result of the community survey and feedback, the Developmental Analysis Report learning activity was added, which encouraged the students to use multiple sources of information for the report, including the reflection papers.

The Developmental Analysis Report emphasized observations and analysis of specific developmental skills such as sensory, motor, perceptual, cognitive, social, and emotional abilities. Following the addition of this assignment, the preschool staff reported that the student's observations were more comparative from week to week rather than just reporting on incidental moments during the service experience. The spring Case Report was then added to continue this experience.

In summary, the assessment process is vital for building, deepening, and evolving the community–academic partnership (Gelmon et al., 2001). The assessment methods used for the Head Start service-learning experience reflect the need to create innovative early childhood education experiences.

CONCLUSION

Service-learning in an early childhood education setting provides a rich environment for OT students to understand, apply, and synthesize human development in the context of children's occupational performance. The Head Start service-learning program described in this chapter creates situations where the student creates meaningful connections between the course and the preschool experience. The assignments and experiences facilitate the student's ability to access deeper reflections and move them from merely acknowledging a reflective thought to critically reflecting, analyzing, and transforming a perspective. Through this service-learning experience, the children, OT students, preschool staff, and academic faculty broaden their perspective of what may be possible in the world (Bronfenbrenner, 1995, 1999; Dunn, Brown, & Youngstrom, 2003).

Dewey (1938) believed that learning is a process, not an outcome involving an evolving interaction of people with their environments. These personal–environmental conflicts transform the person's knowledge and understanding of the world. Learning is optimized when the person is aware and observes the encountered situations, reflects on the situation, and creates meaning and purpose of the situation. The creation of meaning and purpose for learning gives momentum for future action and inquiry. In addition, Dewey (1916) believed that education should reflect humanistic qualities, such as learning for personal growth, to improve the human condition, and to participate in the social fabric of the world. The USP–KenCrest Head Start service-learning partnership captures Dewey's humanistic concepts of education.

REFERENCES

Ash, S. L., & Clayton, P. H. (2004). The articulated learning: An approach to guided reflection and assessment. *Innovative Higher Education, 29,* 137–154.

Bringle, R. B., & Hatcher, J. A. (1996). Implementing service learning in higher education. *Journal of Higher Education, 67*(2), 221–239.

Bronfenbrenner, U. (1995). Developmental ecology through space and time: A future perspective. In P. Moen, G. H. Elder, & K. Luscher (Eds.), *Examining lives in context: Perspectives on the ecology of human development.* Washington, DC: American Psychological Association.

Bronfenbrenner, U. (1999). Environments in developmental perspective: Theoretical and operational models. In S. L. Friedman & T. D. Wachs (Eds.), *Measuring environments across the lifespan.* Washington, DC: American Psychological Association.

Dewey, J. (1916). *Democracy and education.* New York: Macmillan.

Dewey, J. (1938). *Experience and education.* New York: Macmillan.

Dunn, W., Brown, C., & Youngstrom, M. J. (2003). The ecology of human occupation. In P. Kramer, J. Hinojosa, & C. Royeen (Eds.), *Perspectives on human occupation: Participation in life.* Philadelphia: Lippincott, Williams & Wilkins.

Gelmon, S. B., Holland, B. A., Driscoll, A., Spring, A., & Kerrigan, S. (2001). *Assessing service learning and civic engagement: Principles and techniques.* Providence, RI: Campus Compact.

Hohmann, M., & Weikart, D. P. (2002). *Educating young children: Active learning practices for preschool and child care programs,* 2nd edition. Ypsilanti, MI: High/Scope Press.

Ideishi, S. K., Ideishi, R. I., Gandhi, T., & Yuen, L. (2006). Inclusive preschool outdoor play environments. *School System Special Interest Section Quarterly, 13*(2), 1–4.

Kesler-Gilbert, M. (2003). *Teaching towards agency: Exemplary community-based course construction.* Paper presented at West Virginia & Pennsylvania Campus Compact Service-Learning Institute, Morgantown, WV.

Kramer, P., Ideishi, R. I., Kearney, P. J., Cohen, M., Ames, J. O., Shea, G. B., Schemm, R., & Blumberg, P. (2007). Achieving curricular themes through learner-centered teaching. *Occupational Therapy in Healthcare, 21,* 185–198.

Lorenzo-Lasa, R., Ideishi, R. I., & Ideishi, S. K. (2007). Facilitating preschool learning and movement through dance. *Early Childhood Education Journal, 35*(1), 25–31.

Suarez-Balcazar, Y., Muñoz, J. P., & Fisher, G. (2006). A model of university–community partnerships for occupational therapy scholarship and practice. In G. Kielhofner (Ed.), *Scholarship in occupational therapy: Methods of inquiry for enhancing practice* (pp. 632–642). Philadelphia: F.A. Davis.

University of the Sciences in Philadelphia. (2008). Direct-entry master's in occupational therapy program. Retrieved June 25, 2008, from http://www.usp.edu/ot/otdemasters.shtml.

Witchger Hansen, A., Muñoz, J., Crist, P, Gupta, J., Ideishi, R., Primeau, L., & Tupé, D. (2007). Service learning: Meaningful, community-centered professional skill development for occupational therapy students. *Occupational Therapy in Healthcare, 21,* 25–49.

Chapter 10

Community Engagement: A Process for Curriculum Integration

Kimberly Hartmann, PhD, OTR/L, FAOTA

> *"Community engagement is both an art and a skill, and it is an opportunity to help in the community in a caring and compassionate way, while enhancing personal occupational skills. The faculty and students guide, teach, inspire our clients in skills they never dreamed possible to possess. Each session is infused with a sense of purpose, meaning, as well as fun."*
>
> —S.F., Social Worker, Clinical Coordinator of Village of POWER,
> October 2008

Occupations. Defining this term and occupational therapy has been a continual task for members of the occupational therapy profession. In particular, educators need to facilitate student appreciation, examination, and advocacy of occupation and its meaning as a foundation for learning and for the future of professional practice. Occupations have unique meaning to an individual. They contribute to individual and collective identity and provide a framework for how an individual allocates time and resources. Occupations are the primary mechanism toward fostering an individual sense of achievement; collectively, occupations contribute to one's sense of well-being and health (American Occupational Therapy Association [AOTA], 2002).

If understanding the meaning of occupation is critical to becoming a competent occupational therapy professional, then what is best practice in education to provide opportunities for occupational therapy students to experience, internalize, and understand the diversity and richness of occupations? One answer could be in the examination in a term from the *Occupational Therapy Practice Framework: Domain and Process* (AOTA, 2002)—*engagement.*

Engagement in occupation relates to a "commitment made to performance in occupations or activities as the result of self-choice, motivation, and meaning and alludes to the objective and subjective aspects of being involved in and carrying out occupations and activities that are meaningful to the person" (AOTA, 2002, p. 631). Community engagement relates to a commitment to an individual as a part of a relational community and the occupations of the individual in the community. It involves a commitment to the public purposes and aspirations of the community as well as the individual (Holland 1998; Seifer & Connors, 2007).

Moreover, the community's public purposes and aspirations are their occupations, thus connecting the opportunity of engagement in the community to a potential avenue for occupational therapy students to experience occupations.

This chapter focuses on the process for developing service-learning as a method for community engagement for students and faculty to meet the goal of experiencing the breadth and depth of occupations of individuals in community. Thus, community engagement through service-learning provides students with an opportunity to learn the foundations of occupational therapy while providing faculty a novel opportunity to develop scholarship in community engagement.

The chapter will describe the process implemented within a curriculum in a masters' occupational therapy program to meet the goals of the community, students, and faculty for community engagement, learning, and scholarship. The overall process of discovering service-learning is described as: (1) matching service-learning to the mission of the university, and (2) matching the faculty interests to the purposes and aspirations of the community. The process for developing, sustaining, and evaluating service-learning is presented with a final description of the lessons learned and future considerations.

PROCESS

The process of developing a community engagement project began secondary to curricular outcome assessment. Outcome assessment indicated that students were experiencing difficulty understanding the depth and breadth of occupations of groups or systems in the community. This outcome led faculty on a process of discovery of service-learning as a way to meet needs identified by the community and a possible education method to meet the identified need for learning about occupations within the community. Figure 10-1 depicts the major steps that led this program to the development of a service-learning program.

DISCOVERING SERVICE-LEARNING:
THE STARTING QUESTION

Occupational therapy students achieved the course learning outcomes. However, graduate student exit interviews and focus group outcome assessments that were conducted following the final fieldwork experience indicated that students were concerned about their perceived narrow perspective of the definition of *occupation*. A faculty review of the course indicated that readings, writings, video case analyses, and exams were relevant methods of fostering learning. Additionally, feedback from the students on fieldwork Level I indicated that the students were applying the concepts of occupation in

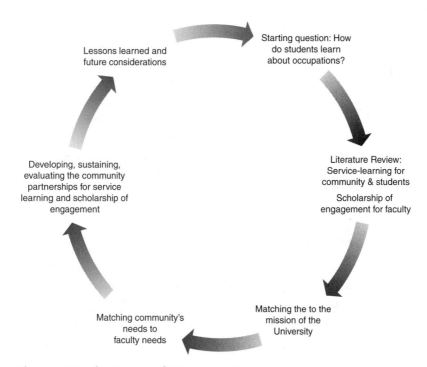

Figure 10-1 The Process of Discovering Service Learning.

the structured fieldwork Level I sites. However, a summary of student interviews and focus groups indicated the following:

1. The students reported that they were unaware of the variations in types of occupations.
2. The students reported that they did not recognize that occupations were still critical to clients and their families even when the client was terminally ill, in a light level of coma, or significantly impaired due to cognitive and/or physical challenges.
3. The students reported feeling limited in the breadth of occupations that may be important to clients as related to the type of community setting where the client lived.

Based on the faculty review process, faculty did not believe that changes in fieldwork Level I would directly facilitate or guide the students to learn more about occupations. What was needed were opportunities to experience being engaged in occupations with individuals within a natural environment, without a therapeutic intervention process. This may be the most appropriate teaching strategy to facilitate student learning about occupation (O'Brien & DiAmico, 2004). However, based on the qualitative student feedback after this approach was instituted, the question remained unresolved: How can students learn about occupations? A review of the literature conducted by the occupational therapy faculty led to the discovery of the powerful potential of service-learning.

LITERATURE REVIEW AND ANALYSIS: CAN IT MEET OUR COMMUNITY AND LEARNING GOALS?

A literature search on the outcomes of community engagement yielded many relevant articles on how to foster student engagement, with the majority of articles focused on service-learning. Within that same literature search, a second body of literature emerged on the scholarship of engagement (Boyer, 1994), which focused on the roles of the faculty in the community and how community-based learning and engagement could be a form of scholarship.

The literature review also included information on service-learning that reflected a multitude of definitions of service-learning (Boyer, 1994; Furco, 1996; Jacoby, 1996; Kraft & Swadener, 1994; Morton & Troppe, 1996; Seifer, 1998). The faculty determined that the occupational therapy program had a number of experiential learning opportunities embedded in the curriculum: hours for volunteerism, over 125 hours of fieldwork Level I (observation experiences in areas of occupational therapy), three one-credit problem-based learning seminars, as well as fieldtrips. However, despite these experiential learning methods, the outcome goal of experiencing occupations of groups, or communities, was not successful, according to the students' feedback.

Therefore, upon review of the literature and the identified problem, the occupational therapy program faculty decided to develop a service-learning program, at the following definition for *service-learning*: "A form of experiential education in which students engage in activities that address human and community needs together with structured opportunities intentionally designed to promote student learning and development" (Jacoby, 1996, p. 5). Therefore, service-learning is both pedagogy and philosophy.

To clarify the components of service-learning, Heffernan's (2002) basic principles of service-learning were adopted:

1. *Engagement* through service-learning projects with a community partner.
2. *Reflection* on the service project with peers and faculty in an informal manner.
3. *Reciprocity*, addressing real community needs.
4. *Dissemination*, whereby outcomes of projects serve as models for new projects and the outcomes of the projects are written and/or presented in a public forum so that others can also build upon the projects.

Engagement was defined by the faculty as the interaction in a collaborative manner with persons and their occupations at the community site. Engagement was an active process and meant to actively participate in the preparation process for the occupation, the development and implementation of activities that could lead to the completion of the occupation, or the active completion of the occupation itself (AOTA, 2002). The occupations were defined by the community partner site, therefore reflecting a need expressed by the community. A faculty supervised the engagement process, with the students doing the actual engagement processes with the community partners.

Reflection questions were designed by the students, faculty, and community partners. All three groups completed a reflection grid in either paper or electronic blog format. Critical reflection, reflecting on practice and in practice, was an essential part of the service-learning process (Eyler, 2002; Schön, 1995; Seifer, 1998) and allowed students to connect the service with the key element of occupation. Questions were constructed in a manner to elicit reflections about the occupations and the context variables that may have influenced the success of the occupations for the individual at the community site. Identified reflection questions that focused the students on occupation included:

1. What occupations were done, and what indicators were observed or discussed that made it evident that the clients were engaged in occupations?
2. How did you know that the occupations were meaningful and unique to the individual?
3. How were the occupations impacted by context variable of the community site, include a reflection on culture, physical, social, personal, spiritual, temporal, and virtual? (AOTA, 2002)
4. What impact or influence did your engagement with the clients have on their achievement of their occupations?
5. How did the community setting impact your engagement with the client in their occupations?

Each faculty member stressed the importance of "intentionally considering the experiences" (Hatcher & Bringle, 1997, p. 153) as those experiences related to the occupations of the community. Faculty also completed the reflection questions and shared their critical reflections after the students completed their reflection. This reciprocity of learning was perceived by the faculty as a powerful tool for critical and ethical reasoning (Greene, 1997), forming observation skills, and developing self-confidence for the students (Furco, 1996; Jacoby, 1996; Seifer, 1998).

The goal of reciprocity became apparent as the students engaged with community members in learning about their occupations. A primary goal for this service-learning model was to develop and nurture community partnerships through engagement in an interactive process to address community occupational needs (Giles & Eyler, 1998; Reardon, 2006; Seifer, 1998). Thus, the goals were already established by the community partners. The reciprocity element was embedded in the relationships among students, faculty, and community members, which resulted in individual and mutual needs being met. In order to keep the reciprocity element clear, a goal form was established for each community partner (see Tables 10-1 and 10-2), based on the model presented by Reardon (2006).

Table 10-1 Goals of the Community Partners: Reciprocity Goal Form.

Community Partner	Goal(s) for Community Partner	Strategies	Expected Outcomes	Dissemination	Community Request for Continuation

RELATING COMMUNITY GOALS TO OCCUPATION

The community partners established the goals of the service-learning; the strategies were programs that were not designed by an occupational therapist, yet these goals and strategies provided extensive opportunities for observation of occupations. Paws to Read used trained dogs to serve as the incentive to young readers to read independently. This strategy provided the occupational therapy students with opportunities to observe instrumental activities of daily living, including the care of pets, communication management, and the psychosocial connections between animals and children that can act as a conduit for social participation and active engagement in a critical area of education—reading.

Kids on the Block Puppet Troupe used child-sized puppets and social scripts to explore and educate children on the inclusion of children with disabilities in everyday life. The highly engaging strategy of puppetry allowed occupational therapy students to observe how children explored the performance skills of children with disabilities through the child-sized puppets. The highly interactive question and answer session following each scripted play revealed insights

Table 10-2 Sample Completed Reciprocity Goal Form.

Community Partner	Goal(s) for Community Partner	Strategies	Expected Outcomes	Dissemination	Community Request for Continuation
Special Education in Public Schools	To provide an environment to encourage independent reading.	PAWS to Read http://www.deltasociety.org/CoPartner.htm	Increase in sustained reading time.	Faculty article Grant funding	Request for the program increased by 125% in year two.
Regular Education	To increase awareness on bullying prevention for young children.	Kids on the Block Puppet Troupe http://www.kotb.com/	Increased awareness of bullying in elementary grades.	Faculty article Replication to more sites	Request for program continued at the same rate in year two.
Police and Fire Departments	To disseminate information on helmet and bicycle safety.	SafeKids http://www.safekids.org/	Community attendance at awareness sessions.	Faculty article Newspaper articles	Request for program doubled in year two.

on the performance skills of children with disabilities and how these skills might alter a child's ability to engage in occupations, especially in education, leisure, and social participation. The scripted answers that occupational therapy students provided to the puppetry audience also promoted an understanding of how children with disabilities performed their activities of daily living in order to be prepared to engage in the everyday activities of children.

Safe Kids, a national program that promotes safety awareness, allowed the occupational therapy students to observe the roles, rituals, and routines of children and families from different settings—urban, rural, and suburban—in daily issues of safety, such as home safety (poison prevention, electrical safety), school safety (walking to school, stranger awareness), and play safety (crosswalks, helmets). Through the use of several intervention approaches, including purposeful activity, education, and advocacy, the occupational therapy students were able to meet the mission of the community partners while using the areas of occupations for children and families as a connection to safety and prevention.

The community partners established the goals and the strategies are common and are available to all disciplines; however, the implementation of the strategies and focused observations of the programs were on the active engagement of the community partners and their constituents in the areas of occupation within community environments. Thus, the programs met Heffernan's (2002) principles of service-learning: engagement, reflection, and reciprocity.

DISSEMINATION

Dissemination of the result and outcomes of the community engagement processes and products was essential in order to: (1) support the continuation of the project and publicly recognize the reciprocal benefits of the project to interested communities and (2) provide venues for the public dissemination of community-engaged scholarship. The building of a continued, sustained interest in the service-learning projects was a natural benefit of the programs. Sharing of information and dissemination of program information through publications, newspaper articles, luncheon receptions on campus, grant awards, and radio interviews were instrumental in sustainability of the programs in the community as well as recognition of the programs on campus.

Faculty were very interested in exploring the concept of service-learning, but with the increasing demands on faculty time, including increased pressure to complete scholarship, there needed to be natural linkages to this necessary area of academia (Holland, 1998). The connection was provided by Calleson, Jordan, and Seifer (2005) through the following statement, which was built upon Boyer's (1994) expansion of the framework for scholarship:

> Community-engaged scholarship reflects this range (referring to Boyer's model of scholarship of discovery—the integration of discovery with application) of faculty work within communities which can apply to teaching (e.g., service learning), research (e.g., community-based participatory research), and service (e.g., community service, outreach, and advocacy). (p. 318)

Several critical factors cause faculty to become involved in service-learning. Faculty members are motivated to contribute to the improvement of society, to promote a positive image of the department, and to provide in-depth educational experiences for the students (Holland, 1998). However, with the demands of the academy, it can be a difficult task to balance the intrinsic motivation of faculty to engage in service while meeting demands for scholarship. The occupational therapy faculty collectively determined that service-learning could constitute scholarship, but they were careful to delineate the requirements and the possible scholarly outcomes that would still foster and maintain a reciprocal collaboration without the service-learning projects crossing over to faculty-based research. The faculty developed the following requirements regarding service-learning scholarship:

1. Faculty must be present on-site at the community partner site.
2. Faculty must be the primary facilitator of any problems or goals (Couto, 2001).

3. Faculty must be the University representative and participate in all phases of the partnership, such as initiation, development of goals and strategies, and methods for maintaining the relationship, critical reflection, and dissolution of the partnership, if necessary (Bringle & Hatcher, 2002).

The following possible scholarly outcomes were identified:

1. Peer-reviewed and peer-adopted articles
2. Applied products that allow for the transfer of the learning through the service to practice, which may include development of policies and procedures, training materials, and resource guides (Aday & Quill, 2000)
3. Grants
4. Clusters of community-based materials, such as community public relations campaigns and presentations or clusters of public communication materials (e.g., newspaper, television, or electronic formats)

The scholarly outcomes needed to integrate the service-learning experiences with the theory and scholarship must be available in the public domain in order to be readily reviewed and critiqued by both the community and the academy (Dodds, Calleson, Eng, Margolis, & Moore, 2003). Whenever possible, the scholarly endeavors should also contain evidence-based statements as to the impact of the service-learning experiences on the community partners, the students, or the interactional process of the two partners (Calleson, Kauper-Brown, & Seifer, 2005; Simpson & Fincher, 1999).

MATCHING SERVICE-LEARNING TO THE UNIVERSITY MISSION

The institution's mission has three areas of focus: excellence in education, sensitivity to students, and a spirit of community. The community value is further defined as the local, national, and global community and the roles of the students within each of these settings (Quinnipiac

University, 2007, p. 11). Therefore, the concept of service-learning for students with faculty simultaneously involved in scholarship of engagement matched the mission. This match allowed for a point of entry for funding, faculty release time, and other pragmatic supports for the service-learning development process (e.g., mailings, purchasing giveaway materials, supplies, and small equipment, if necessary). This match also provided a strong argument that a primary value of the University was being met and, therefore, the publicly disseminated publications, presentations, and products (as previously described) should be evaluated as a form of scholarship in the promotion and tenure process. This concept was approved, and the occupational therapy program was able to move forward with the development of community partnerships. The following University supports were requested and approved based on the defined needs in the literature (Morton & Troppe, 1996): grant writing assistance for equipment, a supply budget, mileage reimbursement for travel to the community sites, and a guest speaker budget. The most important budgetary issue was the approval to include service-learning as part of faculty teaching load. Each faculty was awarded two contact hours as part of their teaching responsibilities devoted to developing, sustaining, and implementing service-learning. This was critical in order to have the university recognize the significant importance of reciprocal community engagement projects.

Ongoing support for service-learning is built into the department operating budget, which is about $4,000 per academic year. Three external grants (from state funding agencies) were received for purchasing equipment for specific projects (Kids on the Block Puppets and Backpack Safety).

MATCHING FACULTY INTERESTS WITH COMMUNITY PARTNERSHIPS

An abundance of community agencies in the area wanted to develop partnerships for service-learning. This quantity of community agencies was certainly a significant challenge to the process of matching the faculty interests with the community needs. However, based on the literature (Holland, 1997; Young, Shinnar, Ackerman, Carruthers,

Table 10-3 Matching Faculty Interests with Community Needs.

Faculty Interests	Community Needs	Community Agency or Projects
Animals	Animal-assisted program in hospice Reading programs in communities with English as a second language	PAWS to Read
School safety	Backpack awareness Anti-bullying programs Walking safety Bicycle safety	AOTA Backpack Awareness Kids on the Block Puppets Safe Kids Connecticut
Sewing	Productive sewing in substance abuse center Sewing for children in foster home placement	Local confidential substance rehabilitation programs
Independent living	Fall prevention education Home safety programs Home rebuilding programs	Safe Kids Rebuilding Together
International occupations	Application of any of the above programs to international sites	Projects were applied to community needs in Barbados

& Young, 2007) the faculty decided to proceed with a modified SWOT (strengths, weaknesses, opportunities, and threats) process to match the faculty with the most appropriate community agency in order to maximize faculty interest, thus increasing sustainability and commitment. The faculty first identified who wanted to embark on the development of service-learning, clarified their interests (professional or personal), and then sought community agencies who had already made their interests known to the University who also matched the faculty member (see Table 10-3). The most critical piece in this step of the process was having the faculty clearly identify their interests, knowing that this element would be critical to meet the time-consuming, collaborative, resource-intensive, communicative process necessary to develop a service-learning project (Lasker, Weiss, & Miller, 2001) on human occupations.

Once faculty involvement was secured and supports were in place from the university, the process of developing the community relationships and embedding student involvement was initiated, and of course continues on a regular basis.

CHALLENGES IN THE MATCHING PROCESS

The primary challenge learned from this experience from a management perspective was sustainability, especially during those periods of the calendar year when students are not available to continue service-learning and when faculty workloads make it difficult to schedule service-learning at those times that are important to the community partners (Eyler, 2002). This challenge continues to exist and needs to be revisited with the development of a new university–community partnership, when new faculty select to facilitate a service-learning experience, and when new students begin the occupational therapy program.

Additional challenges that have occurred when trying to match the missions of the university, occupational therapy department, and the community partner are as follows:

1. The funding structure of each and how that impacts the approval process for money.
2. The administrative structure of each and how that impacts who within the administrative hierarchy needs to be consulted and approval sought when a program is established.
3. The privacy and confidentiality policies for both the community partners and the students.
4. Understanding the mission of the community partner and how that could be met through service-learning that would also allow students to learn through reflection about the occupations of those in the community partnership.
5. Developing pre-service-learning experiences for the students so that they would understand the value of service-learning was

in the mutual partnership and the meeting of the community partner's mission.

6. The pragmatics of scheduling service-learning, which often does not fit into the traditional university class scheduling process and must include travel time, setup time, and reflection process time.

DEVELOPING AND SUSTAINING COMMUNITY PARTNERSHIPS AND STUDENT INVOLVEMENT

Faculty interests were matched with the community agencies who expressed interest in service-learning partnerships. Students were presented with the community needs, the strategies for intervention, and the schedule for the academic semester. Based on this information, the students selected the project that matched their interests and schedules. A modification of the CARE (collaborate, act, reflect, and encourage) model (Cleary, Kaiser-Drone, Ubbes, Stuhldreher, & Birch, 1998) was used to establish the service-learning process, initiate the services, and continue the services each year. The following is an outline of the modified CARE model:

1. Identify and establish rapport.
2. Establish student groups.
3. Students investigate the community agency's mission, goals, programs, and funding sources.
4. Students make hypotheses about the possible occupations of the clients served in the community agency

Collaborate

Faculty, students, and community partners establish rapport and complete the reciprocity goal form (see Table 10-1) to include:

1. Goals/needs of the community partner
2. Goal for the students/University to learn about human occupations
3. Strategies/activities
4. Expected outcomes
5. How outcomes will be evaluated and disseminated

Act

1. Faculty, students, and community partners are trained in and practice the activities and service (e.g., learning the scripts for Kids on the Block puppets, learning how to weigh students and educate students on backpack safety, or learning how to provide public information on home safety).
2. Active engagement by the faculty and students within the natural environments of the community partner.

Reflect

As has been discussed in previous chapters , reflection is a critical piece of the service-learning process. Reflection questions may be focused on the community event, the impact of the community event on the areas of occupation, the interconnections of the context variables and the occupations, or the students' perceptions on the impact of the projects on participants' change in engagement in the areas of occupation.

Encourage

At the end of each semester, the reciprocal goals and outcomes are reviewed and the celebration of student learning, achievement of community goals, and planning for the dissemination of the outcomes are used as tools to encourage the process to continue. Joint celebrations over a meal with both university and community agency administrators facilitates continued discussion and highlights the accomplishment of the community, students, and faculty.

LESSONS LEARNED FROM ONE UNIVERSITY

The lessons learned are vast and immeasurable. However, some key anecdotal points expressed by faculty, community agencies, and students are noteworthy and may prevent potential areas of concern:

1. A community agency may have a mode of operation that is unfamiliar to academia, and bridges must be constructed to communicate in terms that everyone understands.

2. Liability, letters of agreement or understanding, and in some cases contracts, take time to establish and negotiate; expect this process to take longer than you anticipated.
3. Collaboration and mutual goals are essential but may be time intensive.
4. Reflect on boundaries and roles. It is difficult to stay in the role of service without crossing into a therapeutic relationship; make a conscious effort to discuss this with all members of the service-learning process.
5. Plan for those times during a calendar year when students are not available or faculty may not be available, because most community agencies are on a 12-month calendar and may need service-learning to be maintained throughout the year.
6. Every situation can become a learning situation, but the faculty need to be actively engaged with the students in the community in order to experience the situation and reframe, remold, and facilitate the students so that the service-learning is always a teachable moment.
7. Embrace, admire, and enjoy the breadth and depth of human occupations and the power of those occupations to impact health, well being, and quality of life.

SUMMARY AND PLANS FOR THE FUTURE

The service-learning program has been in existence since 2001. Qualitative interviews and focus groups have been the primary forms of measurement of student learning, the reciprocal goal form has been the measure of community achievement, and a variety of dissemination products have been the evidence of scholarship of engagement. However, the occupational therapy program recognizes the need for outcome research on student learning and community satisfaction. As the service-learning programs continue and new ones are developed based on faculty interest and community need, a next step in the process will be developed—outcome measurement.

The element of engagement for faculty, students, and community partners has allowed students to experience human occupations in natural and diverse environments. This experience of engagement in occupations while meeting a community need has allowed for the development of a unique, internalized sense of the power of occupations, not only for students but for faculty as well.

SERVICE-LEARNING WEB SITE RESOURCES

- National Service-Learning Clearinghouse: www.servicelearning. org
- National Service-Learning Partnership: www.service-learning partnership.org/site/PageServer
- New Horizons for Learning: www.newhorizons.org/strategies/ service_learning/front_service.htm
- Campus Contact: www.compact.org/syllabi/

REFERENCES

Aday, L. A., & Quill, B. E. (2000). A framework for assessing practice-oriented scholarship in schools of public health. *Journal of Public Health Management Practice, 6,* 38–46.

American Occupational Therapy Association. (2002). Occupational therapy practice framework. Domain and process. *American Journal of Occupational Therapy, 56,* 609–639.

Bringle, R. G., & Hatcher, J. A. (2002). Campus–community partnerships: The terms of engagement. *Journal of Social Issues, 58*(3), 503–516.

Boyer, E. L. (1994, March 9). Creating the new American college. *The Chronicle of Higher Education, XL*(27), A48.

Calleson, D., Jordan C., & Seifer S. D. (2005). Community-engaged scholarship: Is faculty work in communities a true academic enterprise? *Academic Medicine, 80,* 317–321.

Calleson, D., Kauper-Brown, J., & Seifer, S. D. (2005). Community-engaged scholarship toolkit, community-partnerships for health, from http://www. communityhealthpartnership.com/

Cleary, M. J., Kaiser-Drobney, A. E., Ubbes, V. E., Stuhldreher, W. L., & Birch, D. A. (1998). Service-learning in the third sector: Implications for professional preparation. *Journal of Health Education, 29*(5), 304–311.

Couto, R. A. (2001, Spring). The promise of a scholarship of engagement. *New England Resource Center for Higher Education, Academic Workplace,* 4–7.

Dodds, J., Calleson, D., Eng, G., Margolis, L., & Moore, K. (2003). Structure and culture of schools of public health to support academic public health practice. *Journal of Public Health Management Practice, 9,* 504–512.

Eyler, J. (2002). Reflection: Linking service and learning; Linking students and communities. *Journal of Social Issues, 58*(3), 517–534.

Furco, A. (1996). Service-learning: A balanced approach to experiential education. *Expanding Boundaries: Service and Learning, 1,* 2–6.

Giles, D. E., & Eyler, J. (1998, Spring). A service learning research agenda for the next five years. *New Directions for Teaching and Learning, 73,* 65–72.

Greene, D. (1997). The use of service learning in client environments to enhance ethical reasoning in students. *The American Journal of Occupational Therapy, 51*(10), 844–852.

Hatcher, J. A., & Bringle, R. G. (1997). Reflections: Bridging the gap between service and learning. *Journal of College Teaching, 45*(4), 153–158.

Heffernan, K. (2002). Foundations of service-learning curricula. Campus Compact. Retrieved April 13, 2003, from http://www.compact.org.

Holland, B. (1997, Fall). Analyzing institutional commitment to service. *Michigan Journal of Community Service Learning,* 30–41.

Holland, B. (1998). Factors and strategies that influence faculty involvement in public service. *Journal of Public Service and Outreach, 4*(1), 37–44.

Jacoby, B. (1996). Service-learning in today's higher education. In B. Jacoby (Ed.), *Service-learning in higher education: Concepts and practices* (pp. 3–25). San Francisco: Jossey-Bass.

Kraft, R., & Swadener, M. (1994). *Building community: Service learning in the academic disciplines.* Denver: Colorado Campus Compact.

Lasker, R. D., Weiss, E., & Miller, R. (2001). Promoting collaborations that improve health. *Education for Health, 14*(2), 163–172.

Morton, K., & Troppe, M. (1996). From the margin to the mainstream: Campus Compact's project on integrating service with academic study. *Journal of Business Ethics, 15,* 21–32.

O'Brien, S. P., & D'Amico, M. L. (2004). Scholarship of engagement and service learning: A natural fit in occupational therapy curricula. *Education Special Interest Section Quarterly, 14,* 1–3.

Quinnipiac University. (2007). *Quinnipiac University Catalog, 2007–2008.* Hamden CT: Quinnipiac University.

Reardon, K. M. (2006). Promoting reciprocity within community/university development partnerships: Lessons from the field. *Planning, Practice & Research, 21*(1), 95–107.

Schön, D. (1995, November–December). Knowing in action: The new scholarship requires a new epistemology. *Change, 27,* 26–34.

Seifer, S. D. (1998). Service-learning: Community–campus partnerships for health professions education. *Academic Medicine, 73*(3), 273–277.

Seifer, S. D., & Connors, K. (2007). Community campus partnerships for health: Faculty toolkit for service-learning in higher education. Scotts Valley, CA: National Service-Learning Clearinghouse, from http://www.compact.org/ricompact/content-resources.php#Software.

Simpson, D. E., & Fincher, R. M. (1999). Making a case for the teaching scholar. *Academic Medicine, 74,* 1296–1299.

Young, C. A., Shinnar, R. S., Ackerman, R. L., Carruthers, C. P., & Young, D. A. (2007). Implementing and sustaining service-learning at the institutional level. *Journal of Experiential Education, 29*(3), 344–365.

Chapter 11

Involve Me and I Understand: Differentiating Service-Learning and Fieldwork

Patricia Crist, PhD, OTR, FAOTA

Tell me and I forget.
Show me and I may remember.
Involve me and I understand.

—Chinese Proverb

Historically, the essence of this ancient Chinese proverb has always echoed not only the unique service delivery of occupational therapy in general, but it has also became manifest in our loyalty to field-work education as an important and indispensible aspect in the pro-fessional development of every future entry-level practitioner. Like all other health science professions, occupational therapy has valued some form of practitioner-based apprenticeship as central to injecting students with the ability to translate theory into the realities of everyday practice competence. However, colleges and universities have recently embraced the service-learning approach with incredible swiftness to instill active social justice values, including citizenship, civility, community, and responsibility as a critical aspect in the full development of graduates, particularly at the undergraduate level in higher education.

The goal of this chapter is to compare and contrast service-learning and fieldwork education in occupational therapy to differentiate their practical application and outcomes. However, this is not an easy task, and this chapter will most likely initiate further debate. Regardless, this review cannot be done outside the literature on engaged learning. Thus, a brief review of the major approaches to engaged learning from the broadest models moving to the two that are the specific thesis of this chapter will be provided. Overviews of a variety of engaged learning approaches are provided, including experiential education, community engagement, cooperative education, and service-learning, in order to understand external pressures or opportunities created by these for fieldwork education. The chapter will conclude with specific comparison of service-learning with fieldwork education and provide some guidelines for differentiating the two educational approaches.

Note that specific instructional methods using engaged learning strategies in the classroom, such as mastery or competence-based, problem-based, case-based, and cooperative learning, are beyond the purview of this paper. This chapter focuses on engaged strategies that are useful in naturally occurring ("reality-based") service delivery or practice contexts.

ENGAGED LEARNING OVERVIEW

The purpose of this section is to provide a brief overview of engaged learning from several major models whose focus is to move students from being passive recipients of learning to becoming actively engaged in their own learning process. Information on each model is provided to provide perspectives from each to enhance our understanding of the intent and delivery of service-learning and/or fieldwork education in occupational therapy. The reader is encouraged to read the literature on any one of these opportunities, and the engaged learning resources list at the end of the chapter provides a good starting point.

Engaged learning has the potential to actively integrate three types of thinking advocated as outcomes of educational processes. Fink (2003) specifies the types as:

- Critical thinking—to compare, analyze, and evaluate
- Creative thinking—to design new forms, styles, or programs; to interpret old work in new ways
- Practical/applied thinking—to learn how to answer questions, to make decisions, and to solve problems

Implementing activities to encourage student's development in these three ways of thinking is the foundation for engaged learning.

In an effort to capture researchers' emphasis on desired educational reform in the twenty-first century, Jones, Valdez, Nowakowski, and Rasmussen (1994) succinctly outline the guiding indicators for all engaged learning. Engaged learning includes the following aspects:

- Engaged learners are responsible for their own learning. These learners are strategically and creatively motivated to self-regulate and self-direct their learning.
- Engaged learning is challenging, authentic, and collaborative. Learning activities are sufficiently complex requiring sustained amounts of time and focused attention to be successful. The activities occur in as natural contexts as possible, preferably in the home and workplace.
- Engaged learners continuously assess their acquired learning to ensure that their learning goals are achieved. Performance-based assessment is essential as the student's actual actions,

not paper-and-pencil or oral report, are essential to observe in order to determine that learning has be acquired.

- Instruction uses interactive and generative engagement in a learning environment, preferably as a member of some type of learning or knowledge-building community or group.
- Learners are encouraged to explore and reflect on their applied experiences and discoveries with the physical and interpersonal environment to approximate the cognitive process, critical thinking, associated with a like-minded professional in the specific context.

The goal of engaged learning is to create individuals capable of making significant contributions to the community, practice, and professional knowledge. In applying these guiding indicators, field-work education in occupational therapy would not be considered engaged learning, because the goal for fieldwork is to demonstrate practice competencies and, for the most part, self-direction of learning or even collaboration between fieldwork educator and student are minimized.

Historically, occupational therapy scholars and leaders would reminisce on much earlier work by Donald Schön (1983) regarding reflection-in-action, which initiated our extensive evolution on the development of clinical reasoning in occupational therapy in the late 1980s. Reflections were utilized as a way to enlarge one's clinical reasoning capacities or practice-based critical-thinking processes. The development of clinical reasoning permeates much of occupational therapy education, because the learning outcome of being able to critically learn and effectively use information is more important than the acquisition of a bounded set of facts or skills (Schell & Schell, 2007). However, the use of reflection did not appear in the educational standards for occupational therapy education until nearly 20 years later (Accreditation Council for Occupational Therapy Education, 2006a, 2006b, 2006c).

From these discussions in our profession, interest in evolving approaches to engaged learning in natural contexts has increased rapidly to include, but not limited to, experiential education, including cooperative education and service-learning. It is important to understand each of these educational approaches before discussing the relationship between service-learning and fieldwork education, because they occur within a larger context called *engaged learning*.

Engaged learning, frequently referred to as *experiential education*, is an exciting educational approach because it makes it possible to link teaching, scholarship, and service. Further, it decreases, possibly eliminating, the boundaries between the academy and community. Unlike fieldwork education, engaged learning provides a meaningful approach to building partnerships in which both the education and the community mutually benefit.

EXPERIENTIAL EDUCATION MODEL

Using learning styles as a background, David Kolb (1984) defined the experiential learning theory whereby knowledge is created through the transformation of experience. The learner must first grasp the experience through concrete experience (experiences) and reflective (reflecting) observation, which leads to forming abstract conceptualization (thinking; comprehension) as the basis for transforming this information through active experimentation or testing in new situations (acting; apprehension). Both grasping and transforming experiences are required to maximize learning; however, more recent work describes how adults learn through making meaning of their experiences. Reflections support learning as knowledge is discovered and actions taken; the options are weighed against past learning in order to consider preconceptions, and, ultimately, the unfolding outcomes from the experience. Reflection adjusts the learner's experience and is useful in measuring outcomes. The NSEE (2008) promotes experiential learning for intellectual and ethical development, career exploration and personal growth; and cross-cultural and global awareness, including civic and social responsibility. One occupational therapy program reporting experiential learning as a primary educational method is Keuka College.

The use of reflective learning, originally grounded in experiential education models, is now occurring in fieldwork education (Accreditation Council for Occupational Therapy Education, 2006a, 2006b, & 2006c). However, both occur in authentic environments. The obvious difference is that the focus during fieldwork is on primarily reflective engagement to learn new critical thinking regarding practice and not the collaborative, even generative, engagement through a learning-community challenge, as will be observed later in service-learning.

The following sections provide a brief review of other major experiential-based models used in occupational therapy education: cooperative education, volunteerism, service-learning, and fieldwork education.

COOPERATIVE EDUCATION MODEL

The definition and essential characteristics of the co-op model were approved by the boards of the National Commission for Cooperative Education, the Cooperative Education Association, and the Cooperative Education Division of the American Society for Engineering Education.

Cooperative education, or "the co-op model," is defined as a

> A structured educational strategy integrating classroom studies with learning through productive work experiences in a field related to a student's academic or career goals. It provides progressive experiences in integrating theory and practice. Co-op is a constructive partnership among students, educational institutions and employers, with specified responsibilities for each party. (National Commission for Cooperative Education, www.co-op.edu/aobutcoop.htm)

Work experiences include a formalized sequence of placements in appropriate learning environments that engage the student in increasingly productive work related to career or academic goals. Students are recognized as co-op students and spend 20 to 40 hours per week over an entire semester in learning activities that maximize the outcomes for the student, employer, and curriculum objectives.

The synergy between co-op and fieldwork education is obvious. One difference resonates in the use of the word *employee*. In addition, with the co-op model employer benefits are clearly articulated, in comparison to fieldwork, where employer benefits are viewed as by-products or motivators, not primary drivers. Occupational therapy curriculums with reported engagements in cooperative education include, but are not limited to, Culver-Stockton College, LaGuardia Community College, North Park University, and the University of North Dakota.

VOLUNTEERISM

Service-learning and fieldwork education are not volunteerism. Service-learning is focused on civic engagement that places the community's needs first. Volunteerism is considered a charitable activity grounded in altruism and prosocial behavior, not the formation of reciprocal partnerships, as found in service-learning. Volunteering, including community service, means to "fit-in" and provide service for the existing organization or agency's culture. Learning is secondary and is limited to students gaining a pragmatic understanding of a community agency or service.

SERVICE-LEARNING EDUCATION MODEL

Service-learning is more than an instructional method for student professional development. The notable contribution is that service-learning is foremost a means of addressing community issues and problems. Other chapters in this text have described service-learning more extensively and are to be relied upon for further information. Suffice it here to say that *service-learning* is a structured, community activity where students apply their professional and academic learning to real-world problems or challenges that have been negotiated with a community partner as potentially beneficial or meaningful. Through principle-centered, reciprocal partnerships with the community, students place their professional roles and citizenship in the larger social context by addressing real or authentic life challenges and, oftentimes, social justice issues (Seifer, 1998). The community and the student learn from each other, which simultaneously enriches the learning experience, teaches civic responsibility, and strengthens communities (Learn and Serve: America's National Service-Learning Clearinghouse, 2008). Service-learning is being embraced by occupational therapy education programs in the United States and internationally in such places as the United Kingdom (Sheffeld Hallam) and South Africa (Capetown) (Witchger Hansen, Muñoz, Crist, Gupta, Ideishi, & Tupé, 2007).

FIELDWORK EDUCATION MODEL

Fieldwork education or some other similar practice-oriented learning activity has been a continual requirement in occupational therapy. The goal has been for occupational therapy and occupational therapy assistant students to transform classroom learning about theory, service delivery, skills, and attitudes into entry-level practice competencies. Academic programs have had to meet the educational standards required by the Accreditation Council for Occupational Therapy Education (ACOTE). Further, once an academic program addresses these minimal requirements for every education program, they are able to build upon this foundation through fieldwork or similar learning activities that realize fully their program's philosophy and outcomes.

FIELDWORK EDUCATION AND SERVICE-LEARNING: FROM THEORY TO PRAGMATICS

Three major forces have emerged to provide a rich base for student development, but these have led to confusion in terms of clearly differentiating between *fieldwork education* and *service-learning*. First, as has been outlined previously, education has embraced a rich set of engaged learning methodologies in natural contexts. Innovative educators are morphing these models to fit individual needs, and this has blurred the boundaries between each engaged learning approach. Certainly, like the roots of the Peace Corps in the 1960s in addressing global concerns, the growing social crisis in our country, coupled with the desire for meaningful learning that develops students into committed citizens, educational experiences are moving toward learning approaches that can be used to address community needs.

The second major change has occurred as a direct result of decisions in our profession, as evidenced by observations from this author's experiences as a program director, fieldwork education expert, and leader in the profession for over 30 years. Typically, fieldwork education was directed by an occupational therapist. However, in the 1990s, even with our extensive literature on the importance of mentoring for professional development as occupational therapy practitioners, the lack of a sufficient number of fieldwork placements to meet student demand led to adaptive responses to fieldwork supervisory expectations. Part-time supervisory models by occupational therapy practitioners, and even group supervision models, were utilized to answer demand, as long as some form of continuous supervision was available. In order to encourage student exposure to "emerging areas of practice," part-time fieldwork supervision requirements were being sustained with limited evidence regarding professional development implications beyond anecdotal accounts.

Many of the emerging sites were community-based sites such as homeless shelters, forensics or corrections, day-treatment programs, camps, and so on, providing services for marginalized or underserved populations. Although certainly no one could argue that occupational therapy had the potential to make viable contributions in these settings, few debated the short- and long-term implications of training students with minimal professional role models. Instead, the learning experience was exemplified as innovative education preparing students for new career opportunities. Some would argue that this change was justified or even a controversial cover for addressing the fact that in the late 1980s and early 1990s there was an insufficient number of occupational therapy fieldwork educators to meet the demand for student supervision. Thus, the primary

motive for supporting fieldwork in emerging practice was to extend
the number of viable fieldwork placements to meet student placement demand. Only history will tell us the long-term implications
of this process. However, with part-time, off-site supervision being
used with greater frequency, students found themselves addressing
social justice concerns during fieldwork with increased frequency,
and supervision was moved from direct or ongoing regular observation to student reflection and journaling as the basis for supervisor sessions.

Third, our educational standards reflect academic expectations
that our profession believes must be inculcated into our entry-level
practitioners by the end of their academic experience. As noted earlier, Donald Schön's (1983) work on the development of the reflective practitioner created a major paradigm shift to the area of clinical
reasoning as our profession's approach to understanding critical
thinking. Our 2006 educational standards (ACOTE, 2006a, 2006b,
2006c), in particular, demonstrate the centrality of reasoning as the
basis for service delivery decision-making and the inclusion of reflection as central to developing the reasoning process (ACOTE
Interpretive Guidelines, 2008):

> **Standard B.10.14.** Ensure that the fieldwork experience is de-
> signed to promote clinical reasoning and reflective practice,
> to transmit the values and beliefs that enable ethical practice,
> and to develop professionalism and competence in career
> responsibilities.

Evidence for meeting this standard:

- The program's Level II fieldwork objectives and assessment
  measures demonstrate promotion of clinical reasoning and
  reflective practice.

Both fieldwork education and service-learning processes, along
with the other engaged learning approaches, strengthen the ties between didactic and real-world experiences. Each engaged approach
has components that are very congruent with most academic programs in occupational therapy. Studying each affords a greater understanding of the various potential learning outcomes for our

students. For instance, at Duquesne University students complete almost 12 months of service-learning before beginning fieldwork and seldom see an occupational therapist, except one course instructor who serves as a facilitator. Further, to realize our curriculum model and philosophy, the decision was made that all Level I and II fieldwork must be under the direct, full-time supervision of an occupational therapist to enhance mentoring and modeling for the student's professional development. Another academic program might not make the same decision.

The traditional focus of service-learning elevates its focus within the context of community realties to provide service, whereas fieldwork education occurs in practice settings where professional competence acquisition is the guiding force. Table 11-1 compares the traditions of service-learning with fieldwork education in our profession in terms of philosophy, delivery, student role, and process. As a result, in reality the boundaries of using these two traditions of engaged learning are blurred as a result of our history in fieldwork education.

The implementation of fieldwork education is highly variable today. This is the result of academic programs in occupational therapy creating fieldwork that reflects its specific curriculum philosophy and desired student learning outcomes coupled with the realities of available resources and opportunities. Certainly, one cannot fail to note that learning with "purpose" or "meaning" is highly motivating for students. Fieldwork is purposeful for students, because it is readying them for their career. Likewise, service-learning is motivational, because it creates real results or change, and students are differently motivated when their work is not just a simulation or writing activity but addresses a real need or produces a beneficial resource or utility.

Although occupational therapists by nature are specialists in creative or innovative approaches, evidence is lacking regarding the learning outcomes that result from each of the service-learning and fieldwork education approaches separately or in relationship to each other. Further, the results of learning that combines the essence of both related to the specific professional development of our future

Table 11-1 Comparing Service-Learning and Fieldwork Education.

Service-Learning	Fieldwork
Philosophy or Purpose	
Student-directed partnership with community	Fieldwork educator/site directed
Social justice learning emphasized	OT practical learning emphasized
Community partnership focused[1]	Professional development focused[1]
Delivery	
More process driven (reflection)	More outcome driven (mastery)
Instructor Role	
Partner, coach, or guide for student learning	Direct or authority for student learning
Student Role	
Active, leading role for student anticipated	More passive, follower role
Emphasis on becoming a citizen in the community and world, larger social context[2]	Emphasis on becoming a healthcare professional
Process	
Requires focused reflection	Promotes reflective practice
Community-centered	Education (standards) centered
Needs analysis as basis for action partnerships	Predetermined by school in collaboration with fieldwork educator
Service activity based in mutuality: partnership among community agency, university, educator, student reciprocal, with all involved as learners[1]	Student learns from fieldwork educator and through the experience: one-way learning[1]
Emphasizes engaged citizenship and social change for improved health and quality of life[1]	Emphasizes skill development in health/medical interventions[1]

[1] Hansen, A. M. (2008). A comparison of reflective practice through service learning and fieldwork education: A conceptual approach. Unpublished paper, Duquesne University.

[2] Seifer, S. D. (1998). Service-learning: Community-campus partnerships for health professions education. *Academic Medicine, 73*(3), 273–277.

practitioners has been hypothesized, but has not been demonstrated conclusively. I have had debates with administrators and faculty colleagues about the use of service-learning as producing more of a social welfare or social work perspective than one focused on the essence of occupational therapy as a rehabilitation science.

As mentioned earlier, occupational therapy needs to examine the impact of service-learning, fieldwork education, and the other engaged learning models discussed earlier on professional development outcomes in students' identity as occupational therapy practitioners. The instructional approach must be studied independently of the equally important outcome of using models where students are minimally supervised by occupational therapists. What is the best engaged learning model? What are our intentions for mentoring and modeling natural context experiences that lead to "best educational practices" in the professional development of our students? No doubt, the contention, "Involve me and I understand" is viable in creating learning opportunities.

Ultimately, what are the best curriculum decisions today that will ensure future practitioners will be able emulate to core tenants in the AOTA Centennial Vision for Occupational Therapy in 2017? Engaged learning, especially fieldwork education and service-learning, hold great promise in converting this vision into everyday practice.

> We envision that occupational therapy is a powerful, widely recognized, science-driven, and evidence-based profession with a globally connected and diverse workforce meeting society's occupational needs.

References

Accreditation Council for Occupational Therapy Education. (2006a). *Accreditation standards for a doctoral-degree-level education program for the occupational therapist.* Rockville, MD: Accreditation Council for Occupational Therapy Education.

Accreditation Council for Occupational Therapy Education. (2006b). *Accreditation standards for a master's-degree-level education program for the occupational therapist.* Rockville, MD: Accreditation Council for Occupational Therapy Education.

Accreditation Council for Occupational Therapy Education. (2006c). *Accreditation standards for the occupational therapy assistant.* Rockville, MD: Accreditation Council for Occupational Therapy Education.

Accreditation Council for Occupational Therapy Education. (2007a). *Guide to compliance with the 2006 OT doctoral-degree-level OT standards.* Rockville, MD: Accreditation Council for Occupational Therapy Education.

Accreditation Council for Occupational Therapy Education. (2007b). *Guide to compliance with the 2006 OT master's-level OT standards.* Rockville, MD: Accreditation Council for Occupational Therapy Education.

Accreditation Council for Occupational Therapy Education. (2007c). *Guide to compliance with the 2006 OTA standards.* Rockville, MD: Accreditation Council for Occupational Therapy Education.

Accreditation Council for Occupational Therapy Education. (2008). *ACOTE standards and interpretive guidelines.* Rockville, MD: Accreditation Council for Occupational Therapy Education.

Fink, C. D. (2003). *Creating significant learning experiences: An integrated approach to designing college courses.* San Francisco, CA: Jossey-Bass.

Jones, B., Valdez, G., Nowakowski, J., & Rasmussen, C. (1994). *Designing learning and technology for educational reform.* Oak Brook, IL: North Central Regional Educational Laboratory.

Kolb, D. A. (1984). *Experiential learning: Experience as the source of learning and development.* Upper Saddle River, NJ: Prentice-Hall.

Learn and Serve: America's National Service-Learning Clearinghouse. (2008). What is service learning? Retrieved from http://www.servicelearning.org/what_is_service-learning/service-learning_is/index.php.

National Commission for Cooperative Education. (2008). Retrieved from www.co-op.edu/aboutcoop.htm.

Schell, B. A. B., & Schell, J. W. (2007). *Clinical and professional reasoning in occupational therapy.* Philadelphia: Lippincott, Williams, and Wilkins.

Schön, D. A. (1983). *The reflective practitioner: How professionals think in action.* New York: Basic Books.

Seifer, S. D. (1998). Service-learning: Community-campus partnerships for health profession as education. *Academic Medicine, 73*(3), 273–277.

Witchger Hansen, A. M., Muñoz, J. P., Crist, P., Gupta, J., Ideishi, R. I., & Tupé, D. (2007). Service learning: Meaningful, community-centered professional skill development. *Occupational Therapy in Health Care, 21*(1/2), 25–49.

Engaged Learning Resources List

EXPERIENTIAL EDUCATION

Association for Experiential Education
3775 Iris Avenue, Suite #4
Boulder, CO 80301-2043
www.aee.org

National Society for Experiential Education
C/O Talley Management Group
19 Mantua Road, Mt. Royal, NJ 08061
www.nsee.org

COOPERATIVE EDUCATION

American Society for Engineering Education, Cooperative Education Division
1818 N Street, NW, Suite 600
Washington, DC 20036-247 www.asee.org/activities/organizations/divisions/index.cfm#Cooperative

National Commission for Cooperative Education
360 Huntington Avenue, 384 CP
Boston, MA 02115-5096
www.co-op.edu

Cooperative Education and Internship Association
PO Box 42506
Cincinnati, OH 45242
www.ceiainc.org

SERVICE-LEARNING

Community-Campus Partnerships for Health
UW Box 354809
Seattle, WA 98195-4809
www.depts.washington.edu/ccph (for specific information on occupational therapy, see http://depts.washington.edu/ccph/servicelearningres.html#OccupationalTherapy)

Corporation for National and Community Service
1201 New York Avenue, NW
Washington, DC 20525
www.nationalservice.org

Learn and Serve: America's National Service-Learning Clearinghouse
ETR Associates
4 Carbonero Way
Scotts Valley, CA 95066
www.servicelearning.org

Conclusions and Reflections on Service-Learning in Occupational Therapy Education

Lynn Gitlow, PhD, OTR/L, ATP, Kathleen Flecky, OTD, OTR/L

An essential part of service-learning is reflection. To honor this process, we conclude this book with a commonly used reflection tool for class discussions, journals, and analysis papers to facilitate deeper meaning in service-learning: A What?, Now What?, and So What? reflection. Through contemplation of these three questions, the essence of reflection prior, during, and after a meaningful situation can be delineated.

What? This is a description of the facts or basic topic or issues, a chronology of events, or observations of moments of service-learning. It addresses the answers to the common who, what, when, and where questions. *So what?* This question looks for meaning, analysis, and evaluation of observations or events in service-learning. It entails cognitive processes of analysis and interpretation along with affective processes of feelings, assumptions, and beliefs that impact our thinking. *Now what?* This final question is about future action. How will information be applied to future understanding of facts, events, and issues? How is one called to respond to new situations to apply knowledge, understanding, and skills when faced with similar circumstances in the future (Eyler, Giles, & Schmiede, 1996)? In our teaching together, we have found these questions as important collaborative questions for students, faculty, institutions, and community partners to grapple with throughout our service-learning courses. Genuine engagement occurs with thoughtful reflection by all stakeholders who experience service-learning. Moreover, we can apply these questions to consider how the contributing authors of this book have moved us to reflect on the process of service-learning in occupational therapy education across the United States.

WHAT?

This book has presented both theoretical and practical information related to service-learning and its use as a pedagological tool in occupational therapy (OT) and occupational therapy assistant (OTA) curricula. In reviewing this collection of experiences from a variety of OT and OTA programs, we have learned a great deal about how to apply best practices of service-learning to solving community-based problems. We have also learned about challenges related to implementing this pedagogy and teaching methodology in our educational programs.

In all of the chapters, the definition of *service-learning* that we presented in Chapter 2 is emphasized and service-learning is distinguished from other types of experiential learning, such as fieldwork education or problem-based learning. The contributing authors emphasize the importance of collaboration with community partners in identifying community-based educational opportunities that can simultaneously solve community-identified problems while accomplishing academic outcomes that are necessary as part of OT or OTA educational programs.

We have seen examples of service-learning endeavors that link community service to a variety academic outcomes, including those related to mental health content, group process skills, health promotion, neurobehavioral content grant writing; advocacy skills; and learning about concepts related to the social justice outcomes of occupational therapy. In addition to meeting a wide variety of academic objectives, the programs discussed in this book provide learning opportunities that meet the needs of community members across the lifespan. The variety of programs certainly align with the six practice areas identified as part of the American Occupational Therapy Association's Centennial Vision: mental health; productive aging; children and youth; health and wellness; work and industry; and rehabilitation, disability, and participation (American Occupational Therapy Association, n.d.).

Finally, opportunities to achieve academic outcomes related to understanding social justice, diversity, and the lived experiences of marginalized groups are presented. These outcomes have received particular attention lately in our field, as evidenced by a recent edition of the *American Journal of Occupational Therapy* (January and February 2009)—devoted to this topic. The chapters by Provident and Velde (2009) remind us that these experiences of marginalization and stigmatization are not typically familiar experiences to many occupational therapy and occupational therapy assistant students. Learning about power imbalance, biases, and stigmas in an authentic learning environment provides powerful shifts in students' thinking, as we have seen and has been reported in other service-learning literature cited in previous chapters. This type of learning is critical to achieving the American Occupational Therapy Association's Centennial Vision, which focuses on meeting the occupational needs of society.

SO WHAT?

Since the 1990s, healthcare educators have been challenged to foster future practitioners who exhibit the ability to function with diverse populations in a variety of fast paced, complex healthcare environments. This is even more of a challenge as educators prepare students to become twenty-first-century practitioners (Cook, Irby, Sullivan, & Ludmerer 2006; Institute of Medicine, 2001; Pew Health Professions Commission, 1998). For example, skills such as critical and creative thinking, partnering with communities to provide improvement to the healthcare system; working as members of interdisciplinary teams; emphasizing the social, economic, and political aspects of health care; and teaching students how to demonstrate caring, ethical, and culturally sensitive practices have all been cited as important for healthcare providers of the future (Cook, Irby, Sullivan, & Ludmerer, 2006; Flecky & Gitlow, 2006; Institute of Medicine, 2001; Pew Health Professions Commission, 1998).

Additionally, we have been urged to reflect on our roots of engaging in meaningful occupation by theorists and leaders in our field (Clark, 2006). Despite these calls in the larger healthcare environment, as well as in occupational therapy, we hear no shortage of concerns that practitioners are not prepared for practice and that occupation is still not being infused into our practice (Nielson et al., 2005). Moreover, challenges to society in general regarding human rights and inequities and disparities remain large on the global radar screen. All of these factors present a challenge—to accomplish our Centennial Vision of upholding our social contract to ensure that all people, communities, and populations can engage in the occupations of their choice. Could it be that educational practices currently in place are not providing the context for learning these twenty-first-century skills? In Chapter 11, Crist challenges us to think about fieldwork versus service-learning as means to accomplish these educational goals.

Further questions have been asked throughout this book regarding how we engender attitudes of responsible citizenship, social justice and solidarity in community in our students?. How do we provide students with opportunities to reflect and engage in the ethics of practice that align with community practice and community needs? How do we engage students in solving community problems and understanding the lived experience of those who experience inequities and disparities? We believe that service-learning certainly is worth exploring as an educational pedagogy capable of educational opportunities in context and in community with others served, underserved or unserved by occupational therapy.

NOW WHAT?

Although it appears that service-learning has value for meeting educational outcomes, one of the challenges in infusing service-learning into higher education curricula is the perception of faculty and institutions of service-learning in particular, and the scholarship of teaching and learning in general as being recognized as a scholarly endeavor. We have noted in the chapter by Hartmann strategies that characterize service-learning as scholarship. Additionally, literature cited throughout this book suggest that not only is service-learning effective pedagogy (Gitlow & Flecky, 2005; Greene, 1997), but also examine the outcomes of service-learning programs on the individuals and the community as more educational and community research advances.

It is important to note how many of the educational programs included in this book report that the mission of their institutions supports their service-learning endeavors. This is identified as an important aspect of successful service-learning experiences (Eyler & Giles, 1996), and Crist identifies the rapid growth of service-learning programs in faith-based schools. It will be notable to see whether this growth continues as we now face serious social, economic, and spiritual problems that cannot be solved by looking to the past or with our current institutional solutions. Scharmer (2009) states that change will come from the future as it emerges rather than from the past or present. We believe that community-based service-learning experiences can emerge from the future. This is an area ripe for scholarship, and we encourage you to investigate questions like this and others as you pursue service-learning experiences.

Will service-learning experiences enhance our future practitioners' abilities to meet the mandate of occupational therapy to enable *all* people, communities, and populations to achieve health by engaging in meaningful occupation (American Occupational Therapy Association,

2008)? Is it possible to harness the power of our communities in concert with our educational programs to educate future practitioners in how to meet the healthcare and occupational needs of *all* people, communities, and populations? Will service-learning enhance our ability to become a powerful globally connected evidence-based profession consisting of a diverse workforce that is focused on meeting the occupational needs of all? These are the questions that the educator authors have addressed in this book in an effort to make education purposeful, relevant, and meaningful within a larger community. We hope the resources in this book will help us all reflect more thoughtfully on these questions as occupational therapy educators.

REFERENCES

American Occupational Therapy Association. (2008). Occupational therapy practice framework: Domain and process, 2nd ed. *American Journal of Occupational Therapy, 62*(6), 627–630.

American Occupational Therapy Association. (n.d.). Practice areas: Occupational therapy practice areas for the 21st century. Retrieved online January 26, 2009, from http://www.aota.org/Practitioners/PracticeAreas.aspx.

Clark, F. (2006). Moving forward: We have the vision, now let's make it happen. Retrieved online September 29, 2008, from http://www.aota.org/News/Centennial/Background/36569.aspx.

Cook, M., Irby, D., Sullivan, W., & Ludmerer, K, (2006). American medical education 100 Years after the Flexner Report. *New England Journal Of Medicine, 355*(13), 1339–1344.

Eyler, J., Giles, D. E. Jr., & Schmiede, A. (1996). *A practitioner's guide to reflection in service-learning: Student voices & reflections.* Nashville, TN: Vanderbilt University.

Flecky, K., & Gitlow, L. (2006, April). *Preparing students for messy practice: Critical reasoning and reflection through service-learning.* American Occupational Therapy Association Annual Meeting, Charlotte, NC.

Gitlow, L., & Flecky, K. (2005). Integrating disability studies concepts into occupational therapy education using service learning. *American Journal of Occupational Therapy, 59,* 546–553.

Greene, D. (1997). The use of service learning in client environments to enhance ethical reasoning in students. *American Journal of Occupational Therapy, 51,* 844–852.

Institute of Medicine. (2001). *Crossing the quality chasm: A new health system for the 21st Century.* Washington, DC: National Academies Press.

Nielson, C., Youngstrom, M. J., Glantz, C., Henderson, M. L., Richman, N., Roley, S. S., Duran, G., & Peterson, M. (2005). The American Occupational Therapy Association report to the executive board: Ad hoc workgroup on implementing occupation based practice. Retrieved online January 15, 2009, from http://www.aota.org/News/Centennial/AdHoc/41327/41346.aspx.

Pew Health Professions Commission. (1998, December,). *Recreating health professional practice for a new century. The fourth report of the Pew Health Professions Commission.* San Francisco: The Center for the Health Professions, University of California.

Scharmer, C. O. (2009). *Theory U: Leading from the future as it emerges. The social technology of presencing.* San Francisco: Berrett-Kohler.

Index